Progress in Clinical Biochemistry and Medicine

C. I. Grossmann, G. A. Roselle

The Control of Immune Response by Endocrine Factors and the Clinical Significance of Such Regulation

W. Trager, M. E. Perkins, H. N. Lanners

Malaria Vaccine

A. Rubinstein, J. R. Robinson

Controlled Drug Delivery

A. Hubbuch, E. Debus, R. Linke, W. J. Schrenk

Enzyme — Immunoassay: A Review

AKADEMIE-VERLAG BERLIN

Progress in Clinical Biochemistry and Medicine

Control of Immune Response by Endocrine Factors

Malaria Vaccine

Controlled Drug Delivery

Enzyme-Immunoassay

With Contributions by
E. Debus, C. J. Grossmann, A. P. Hubbuch,
H. N. Lanners, R. Linke, M. E. Perkins,
J. R. Robinson, G. A. Roselle, A. Rubinstein,
W. J. Schrenk, W. Trager

With 45 Figures

Akademie-Verlag Berlin

Die Originalausgabe erscheint im Springer-Verlag Berlin · Heidelberg · New York · London · Paris · Tokyo als Volume 4 der Schriftenreihe Progress in Clinical Biochemistry and Medicine

Vertrieb ausschließlich für die DDR und die sozialistischen Länder

Erschienen im Akademie-Verlag Berlin, DDR-1086 Berlin, Leipziger Straße 3—4

ISBN 3-540-16955-5 Springer-Verlag Berlin · Heidelberg · New York
ISBN 0-387-16955-5 Springer-Verlag New York · Heidelberg · Berlin
ISBN 3-05-500379-9 Akademie-Verlag Berlin

Lizenznummer: 202 · 100/512/87
Printed in the German Democratic Republic
Gesamtherstellung: VEB Druckerei „Thomas Müntzer“, 5820 Bad Langensalza
LSV 2015
Bestellnummer: 763 733 2 (3078/4)
09800

Editorial Board

Table of Contents

The Control of Immune Response by Endocrine Factors and the Clinicial Significance of Such Regulation

Charles J. Grossmann, Ph. D.[1,2,3] and Gary A. Roselle, M. D.[1,4]

The immune response has been shown to be under the control of a variety of factors including hormones from the pineal, pituitary, thymus, gonads, adrenals, and thyroid. Regulation of these substances by hormonal axes can account for the observed differences in immune responses between sexes as well as affect the onset, course and clinical outcome of disease processes. Fluctuation in hormonal levels resulting from changes in the light-dark cycle may also explain variation in immune response reported in man and experimental animal models. Because of the great volume of diverse publications dealing with hormones and the immune response, and the medical significance of their interactions, we have concisely summarized the pertinent material. While the hormonal regulation of immune function is already proving to be an important area for research, it is expected that within the next few years the interactions between endocrine, neural and immune systems will be even more widely studied.

[1] Research Service and Medical Service, Veterans Administration Medical Center, Cincinnati, OH/U.S.A.

[2] Department of Physiology & Biophysics, College of Medicine, University of Cincinnati, Cincinnati, OH/U.S.A.

[3] Department of Biology, Xavier University, Cincinnati, OH/U.S.A.

[4] Division of Infectious Diseases, Department of Medicine, University of Cincinnati, Cincinnati, OH/U.S.A.

1 Introduction to the Immune System

Although the body is surrounded by a polluted external environment, the human immune system is responsible for protecting it from attack by pathogenic microorganisms as well as other foreign cells and substances. In order to specifically recognize and eliminate foreign invaders, the immune system adoptively responds to the invading organism (or antigen) with great specificity. After this primary immune response is completed, any subsequent challenge with the same antigen will generate

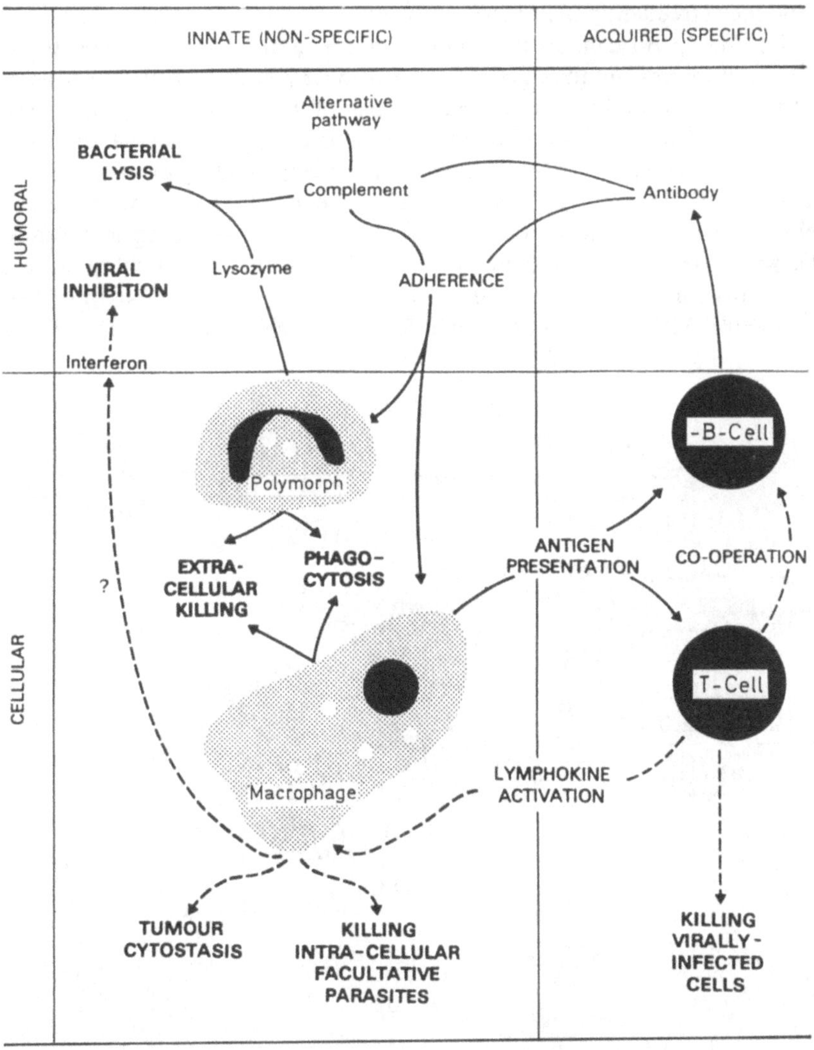

Fig. 1. This is a simplified scheme to clarify the interactions taking place between components of the innate and specific immune systems. Reactions which are influenced by T lymphocytes are indicated by the broken lines. (Developed with permission from Playfair JHL 1974 BRIT MED BULL 30:24)

a secondary immune response resulting from the long term memory retained by memory cells in this system [1-6].

In humans, as in other vertebrates, the immune system (Fig. 1) can be subdivided into the nonspecific or innate immune system and the specific or acquired immune system. The nonspecific immune system encompasses all reactions which are not directly dependent on an antigen challenge. These include inflammatory responses, phagocytosis, and certain aspects of the complement protein interactions [1-6]. The specific immune system involves reactions of the thymus derived. (T) cells and Bursal derived (B) cells (although in humans no Bursa is present and B cells originate in some other location such as the bone marrow, liver or gastrointestinal tract) [1-6].

B cells, and more frequently their progeny, plasma cells, are responsible for manufacturing and secreting proteins called immunoglobins and as such are said to be mediators of the humoral immune system. Activation by host exposure to foreign materials called antigen usually results in phagocytosis of the antigen by macrophages, which then degrade this material and present the remaining antigenic determinants to clones of B cells located in the lymph nodes and spleen. Binding of the antigenic determinant to the B clone cell is accomplished through interactions with surface immunoglobin receptors on the B cell. The clones undergo maturation to produce plasma cells which secrete immunoglobin (or antibody) into the circulation [1-6]. These immunoglobin molecules, which are a class of glycoprotein composed of two heavy chains (50,000 MW each) and two light chains (25,000 MW each) (Fig. 2) are

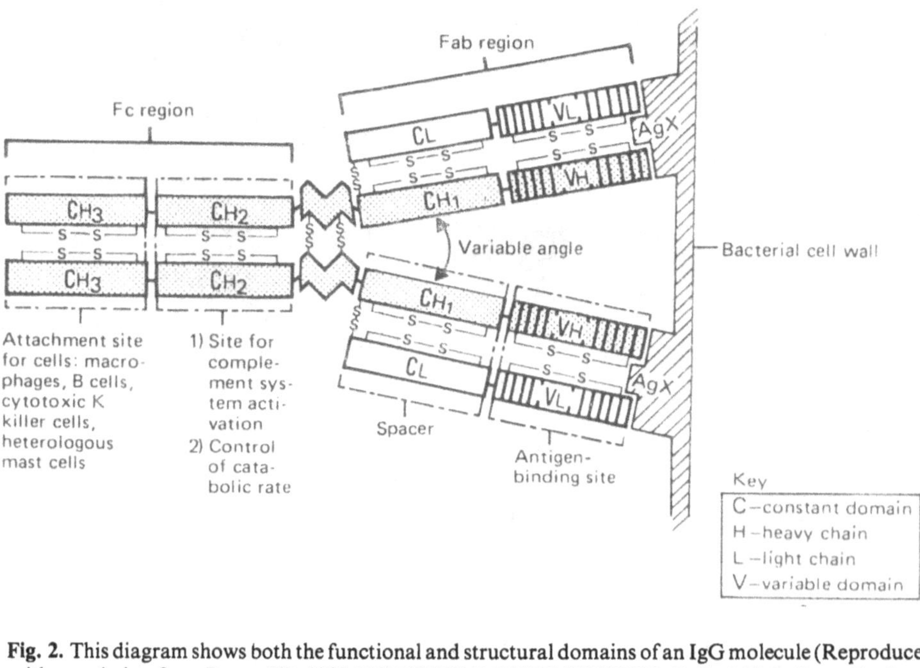

Fig. 2. This diagram shows both the functional and structural domains of an IgG molecule (Reproduced with permission from Bowry TR 1980 IMMUNOLOGY SIMPLIFIED, Oxford Univ Press, England, p. 25)

able to recognize and specifically bind to the stimulating antigen to form an antigen-antibody complex. The formation of this complex then triggers a series of events, (including phagocytosis by polymorphonuclear granulocytes and macrophages, and activation of the classical complement pathways) which lead to the elimination of the antigen from the system. Memory B cells are produced during clonal formation which are programmed to respond to any further stimulation by the original antigen. Such memory cells can rapidly undergo clonal formation and secrete large quanities of immunoglobin [1-6].

As has been described earlier, Thymus-derived lymphocytes (T cells) are mediators of another form of specific immunity known as cell-mediated imunity. Cell-mediated reactions are commonly defined as those immunological responses in which the lymphoid tissues develop a specific cell-mediated defense against foreign antigen [1-6]. Like the reactions involving B cells, T-cells bind antigen first processed by macrophages. Such thymus-dependent antigen has been reported to be principally, but not exclusively, associated with the surface of pathological cells (as for example virally infected cells or cancer cells). The macrophage processed antigenic determinants are presented to T cell clones located in the lymph nodes and spleen and bind to deeply buried T cell surface receptors [1-6]. Binding of the antigenic substance to the specific T-cells produces patching and capping of the receptor antigen complexes and stimulates clonal formation. The progenitor T-cells generated consist of various physiological classes, including killer or cytotoxic T-cells, helper T-cells, suppressor T-cells and memory T-cells [1-6].

Helper and suppressor T-cells regulate B cell production of immunoglobins and assist in the control of tolerance to self antigens. Memory T-cells (like memory B cells) remain in an inactive state for years in the body and, if re-exposed to antigen, rapidly form clones of active T-cells. Killer or cytotoxic T-cells bind to target cell surface antigen and are stimulated to release various substances called lymphokines which possess a variety of functions including the attraction and activation of macrophages, inhibition of viral replication (by interferon) and direct destruction of target cells through alterations of target cell membrane integrity. Such T-cell mediated responses include allograft rejection, allogeneic (graft vs host) disease, and delayed hypersensitivity and, ultimately lead to elimination of the foreign material from the system [1-6].

2 Hormones and Their Mechanisms of Action in the Immune System

Hormones fall into various categories depending on their molecular structure. In the immune system, both steroid hormones and peptide hormones have been reported to regulate function [7-14], although it would not be surprising to learn that other hormones (prostaglandins, amines) could exert major effects as well.

2.1 Mechanism of Action of Steroids and Peptides

The mechanism of action of steroid and peptide hormones in the immune system is similar to that reported in other body tissues. Of paramount importance is the observation that, for any hormone to have an effect, the target tissue must possess receptors specific for this hormone [15-18].

2.1.1 Steroid Hormones

In the case of steroids, the receptors are located in the cytoplasmic fraction and upon binding with the steroid ligand translocate into the nucleus where the hormone receptor complex regulates protein synthesis [15-18].

In the immune system, reticuloendothelial cells of the thymus have been reported to contain receptors for estradiol, dihydrotestosterone, cortisol and progesterone [19-31] while reticuloendothelial cells of the Bursa have been shown to possess receptors for estradiol, dihydrotestosterone, and progesterone [32]. In many studies, steroid receptors for estradiol and dihydrotestosterone have not been identified in the thymic-derived T-cell [19, 20, 24, 28, 30] or Bursa-derived B-cell [32]. However, some studies have reported that such receptors are present in T-lymphocytes [25, 27, 31]. The ability of some investigators to demonstrate the presence of receptors in lymphocytes, while others cannot, may be due to sensitivity of these assays. However, it has been reported that estradiol treatment decreased the large lymphoid cells of the outer thymic cortex [57] and further, that size (and therefore age) of the thymocyte was correlated with presence or absence of estrogen receptors [27]. Large immature lymphoblast cells were shown to possess receptors, while small, mature and immunologically functional thymocytes did not contain receptors [27].

The fact that receptors for sex steroids are present in the reticuloendothelial maxtrix of the thymus, as well as in immature lymphoblasts, suggests that steriods may regulate both immature lymphoblast development and immunological function of the mature thymocytes. Results obtained from many studies to be described later in this chapter support the view that sex steroids functioning through the reticuloendothelial thymic steroid receptors regulate the release of thymic hormones, which alter immune response of thymic-derived lymphocytes.

Glucocorticoids on the other hand are known to function through direct receptor interactions at the level of the thymocyte, as well as the thymus reticuloendothelial cell [33-39]. Bursa of chicks has also been reported to possess glucocorticoid receptors which bind dexamethasone, but the receptors were predominantly localized to the lymphoid fraction [32]. The possibility that receptors for both sex steriods and glucocorticoids are located in the same thymic cell is supported by the observation that castration, which stimulates thymic cell hypertrophy and hyperplasia, increases the number of cortisone sensitive cells [40]. Furthermore, during pregnancy in mice, thymic involution and atrophy takes place along with a reduction in thymocytes located in the cortex, while the steroid-resistant medullary thymocytes remain unchanged [41-43]. These cortical thymocytes must contain steroid receptors in order for them to manifest steroid sensitivity and, because they are also probably the glucocorticoid-sensitive cells which have been reported to increase as a result of castration [40] proves that one type of thymic cell contains steroid receptors for both sex steroids and glucocorticoids.

2.1.2 Peptide Hormones

While steroids acting directly through receptors at the level of the immature lymphoblast could conceivably alter lymphoblast development, thymic hormones (Fig. 3) released from the reticuloendothelial thymic matrix are also known to alter thymocyte development as well as function [7–11]. Such thymic hormones, isolated, purified and characterized by Alan Goldstein's laboratory [12,44,45] possess structures with molecular weight in the range of 3,000–8,500 (thymosin α_1: 3108, thymosin α_7: 2,200, thymosin B_1: 8,451, thymosin B_3: 5,500, thymosin B_4: 4,982) [12].

In the case of both peptide and protein hormones (as well as for many biogenic amines), primary interaction with a membrane-bound receptor initiates a series of reactions to activate adenyl cyclase which then forms the second messenger cAMP [46,47]. In the case of thymosin Fraction 5, the second messenger has been shown to be cyclic GMP [48] but the thymic hormone is probably also working through membrane bound receptors. This is supported by the recent report of Garcia et al. [49] who demonstrated the presence of thymosin α_1 receptors on thymocyte membrane.

Other non-thymic protein or peptide hormones may also exert direct effects on lymphcytes by binding to specific lymphocyte membrane receptors. One example is

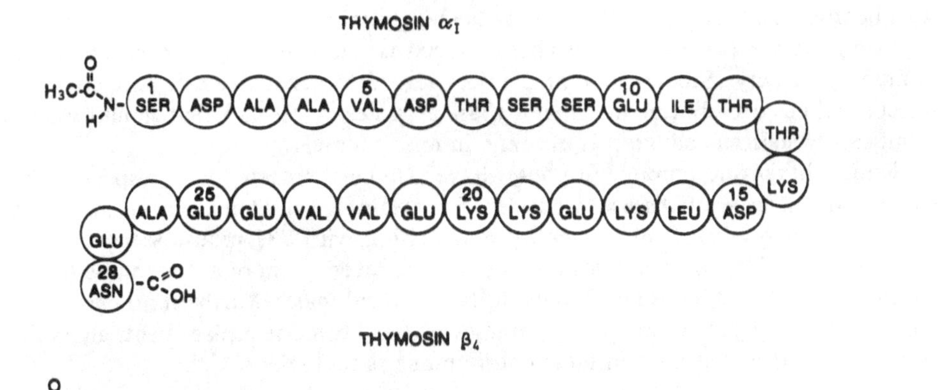

Fig. 3. Amino acid sequences of thymosin α_1 and thymosin B_4. Reproduced with permission from Low TLK, Thurman GB, Zata MM, Hu SK, Goldstein AL 1981 ADVANCES IN IMMUNOPHARMACOLOGY, Pergamon Press, England, p. 69

somatotropin (growth hormone, GH), which has been reported to bind specifically to GH receptors present on the membranes of various types of lymphocytes [50, 51]. T and B lymphocytes have also been shown to possess both insulin and glucagon membrane receptors which are induced on activated lymphoblasts [52–56].

The observation that insulin and glucagon receptors are only present in lymphoblasts undergoing transformation [52–56] is strikingly similar to the report of estrogen receptors only present in lymphoblast cells but not in small lymphocytes [27]. The appearance of these receptors at the time of lymphoblast transformation implies that certain steroids, peptides and protein hormones may play a significant role in lymphocyte maturation and function.

3 Differences in Immune Response Between Males and Females

In females, circulating levels of the immunoglobins (Ig) classes G, M and A exceed those found in males [40, 58–63], and the fluctuating levels of uterine IgA and IgG positively correlate with the circulating levels of estradiol [64, 65]. This elevated response in females has been demonstrated in vitro with the plaque-forming cell (PFC) assay [66] and involves an increase in both IgM PFC and IgG PFC [67, 68]. In studies utilizing mice as the experimental model, females generated a greater and more sustained primary and secondary humoral immune response than did males when challenged with bovine serum albumin (BSA) [69] or hemagglutinin [70].

Skin graft rejection time has also been utilized as a measure of in vivo cell mediated immune reactivity. Studies in inbred mice have demonstrated that skin allograft rejection times are shorter in females than in males [71, 72], and that gonadectomy significantly shortens allograft reject time in male animals [72].

Dimorphic sexual immune responses have also been reported with respect to the cause and outcome of disease processes. For example, adult male mice are more susceptible than adult female mice to innoculation with S37 mouse sarcoma [73, 74] while female NZB mouse hybrids develop a more severe form of autoimmune thyrocytotoxicosis [75] and lupus (7679) then do NZB hybrid males. Furthermore, gonadectomy of NZB hybrid strain animals, along with sex hormone replacement, alters the onset and course of disease in these autoimmune pathologies [75–79].

4 Effects of Gonadectomy, Adrenalectomy and Sex Hormone Replacement on Immune Response

Thymic involution is a normal consequence of the hormonal changes that take place in many mammallian species at puberty. In prepubertally gonadectomized animals, however, thymic involution is delayed and thymic hypertrophy is produced [8, 20, 80–83]. Postpubertal gonadectomy induces thymic hypertrophy with maximal size being obtained by one month after surgery [20, 81, 82] (Fig. 4). An increase in mass of the peripheral lymph nodes and spleen has also been reported to take place in gonadectomized animals [82, 84, 85], although synchronous thymectomy and gonadectomy abrogated the lymph node enlargement that followed castration alone [82], further suggesting a hormonal link between thymus and gonads. Examination of castration-induced enlarged thymus glands utilizing histological techniques demonstrated cellular hyperplasia and hypertrophy in both cortex and medulla [20,82], destruction of thymic lymphocytes, atrophy of the thymic lobules, and increased fat content [81].

Treatment with estradiol [20,81], estrone [81] or testosterone [20,24] has been shown to reduce this castration-induced thymic enlargement, but these steroids are also effective in reducing thymic weight in normal animals. Treatment with gonadotropic hormone [86] has also been reported to decrease thymic size, presumably because it stimulates increased steroid production from the gonads.

Along with the effects on thymic architecture, gonadectomy has also been shown to stimulate thymic cell blast transformation in culture. Thymic cells exposed to serum prepared from gonadectomized male rats underwent a five-fold increase in mitogen-induced DNA synthesis with respect to controls [7-9], while adrenalectomized serum stimulated thymic cell blastogenesis seven-fold [7-9] and combined gonadectomized-adrenalectomized rat serum stimulated thymic cell blast transformation ten-fold [7-9]. This stimulatory effect of gonadectomized serum was abrogated in thymectomized animals, indicating that a thymic hormone under the control of gonadal steroids was involved [7-9].

It has been reported that gonadectomy in mice increased antibody production to the antigens oxazolone and sheep red blood cells, and that skin allograft rejection was accelerated [87,88]. Furthermore, in this castrate mouse model, skin graft rejection was depressed by treatment with androgen [87,88] and, finally, in castrate plus thymectomized mice, the skin graft rejection response was not accelerate [87,88]. Additional support for the depressive effect of sex steroids on immune function can be found in studies where gonads have been transplanted into male and female recipients [72].

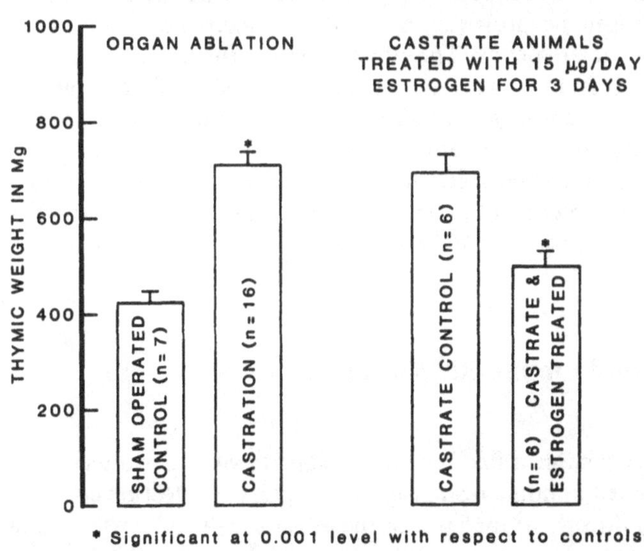

Fig. 4. Alterations in thymic weight resulting from castration and estrogen treatment. Castrate animals were treated with estradiol at a concentration of 15 μg/day for 3 days. (Reproduced with permission from Grossmann CJ, Sholiton LJ, Blaha GC, Nathan P 1979 J STEROID BIOCHEM 11:1241)

Taken together, these results imply that sex steroids depress the cell-mediated immune response, and further supports the hypothesis that thymic hormones are involved.

As has been previously mentioned, in females the circulating levels of IgG, IgM, and IgA exceed those found in males [40, 58-63], and anitbody response to antigen challenge at least for certain antigens is elevated in females over males. For example, polio antigen [63], ascites sarcoma antigen [70], or red blood cell antigen [92,93] stimulate higher titers of antibody in females vs. males. Furthermore, estrogen treatment has been shown to stimulate antibody production [92-94], while gonadectomy has been reported to variously depress [94], elevate [70, 85], switch classes of immunoglobin [85], or have no effect [84, 87, 88, 95].

Two pertinent observations have been made which may account for the higher levels of immunoglobin in females than in males. Firstly, certain antibody-forming genes are located on the "X" chromosome [95, 96], and secondly, estrogen has been shown to increase the proliferative response in spleen and lymph nodes to antigen [97] and to inhibit suppressor T-cell activity which, in turn, enhances B-cell maturation and thus antibody production [7-9, 98].

Gonadectomy has also been shown to alter expression of various pathologic disorders. For example, reactivity of castrate mice to graft vs. host disease (where transplanted immunocompetent donor lymphocytes attack an immunocompromised recipient) is markedly increased [87]. In castrate mice, the induction of methylcholanthene tumors is delayed with respect to non-castrates [84], presumably because gonadectomy stimulated immune surveillance. On the other hand, spontaneous leukemia in AKR mice is increased by gonadectomy, possibly due to thymic hypertrophy, resulting in an increased population of lymphocytes at risk of malignant transformation [84].

In hamsters, gonadectomy at three to four weeks of age results in a lower incidence of Ad 12 tumors and estrogen or progesterone treatment increases tumor onset significantly more in males than females [89]. The effect of steroid treatment on increased tumor incidence may result from either a depression in the cell-mediated immune response, and thus a decrease in tumor surveillance, or it may be due to a direct affect of the steroid on Ad 12 transformation of hamster cells [89, 90]. However, when a non-hormone dependent tumor such as the HeLa cell line is grown in mice, treatment with estrogen enhances tumor growth and inhibits tumor rejection [91] suggesting that a depression in cell mediated immunity is taking place.

5 Effect of Estrogens on Immune Responses

Estrogenic steroids have been demonstrated both in vivo and in vitro to exert a strong depression on the cell-mediated immune response. This depressive effect by estrogen is thought to function both directly at the level of the effector T-lymphocyte [27] and indirectly at the level of the reticuloendothelial thymus cell where thymic hormones are elaborated [7-11]. Thymocyte subsets mediated by circulating thymic hormones have been reported to depress cutaneous delayed hypersensitivity reactions in various animal models [99, 101], as well as suppress or delay rejection of tissue transplants [102].

To account for this immune depression, one need only look at the response of the effector T-lymphocytes in the presence of estrogen. In a study in which NMRI female mice were treated with diethylstilbestrol (a non-steroidal estrogenic compound), spleen lymphocytes showed a significantly depressed response to the mitogens concanavalin A (Con A) or bacterial lipopolysaccharide [103] and peripheral lymphocytes in these animals were decreased in number [103, 104]. Estrogen treatment has also been reported to decrease the natural killer cell activity in mice, which is mediated by small T-lymphocytes [105], and to inhibit the release of thymic hormones in rats, resulting in a reduction in blastogenic transformation of PHA and Con A activated T-lymphocyte subpopulations in vitro [7-11]. Furthermore, blastogenic transformation of PHA activated T-lymphocytes is depressed in women taking oral contraceptives containing either conjugated estrogen alone or conjugated estrogen plus medroxyprogesterone [106].

The onset and course of cancer has also been reported to be altererd by estrogen treatment. For example, the PHA-induced mitogenesis of peripheral blood lymphocytes (the majority of which are probably T-lymphocytes) is depressed in patients with prostatic cancer who are receiving estrogen therapy [107]. Estrogens have also been implicated in suppression of tumor-associated immune responses to malignant prostate or breast cancer in humans [108, 109], along with the development of certain sex-related forms of chemically-induced cancer [110, 111].

The ability of estrogens to promote malignant transformation could reside in either of two mechanisms of action which may act independently or in conjunction. Either the steroids may function directly on normal cells to cause them to metamorphosize into cancer cells, or the steroids may permit carcinogenic development by depressing surveillance of the cell-mediated immune system.

In a number of studies, it is difficult to differentiate between those two mechanisms of action because the experimental cancers are hormone-dependent [111, 115]. However, the Hela tumor is non-hormone dependent and in estrogen-treated female mice Hela tumor growth was prolonged compared to male or female controls or to estrogen-treated males [91]. This finding suggests that sex steroids can depress the immune mechanisms necessary for anti-cancer surveillance. Since hormonal therapy is commonly utilized in treatment of certain forms of cancer, it would appear that in some cases the palliative effects may be countered by a reduction in host responsiveness to malignant neoplasms and underlying infectious agents which may then contribute to the deaths in cancer patients [107, 109].

Parasitic protozoan infections such as those produced by *Toxoplasma gondii* are also inhibited by the cell-mediated immune system. In both guinea pigs and mice, it has been reported that gonadectomy increases resistance to those infectious agents, while treatment with synthetic estrogen results in elevated mortality [116, 117]. These findings lend further support to the suggestion that estrogens depress cell-mediated immune function.

A variety of immunologic disorders have been associated with estrogen, as evidenced by a disproportionate number of women compared to men with specific diseases linked to abnormalities of host response. Perhaps the most notable and well-studied malady of this type is Systemic Lupus Erythematosus (SLE). In this disease, the ratio of women to men is approximately 9:1, with alterations of estrogen metabolism seen in these female patients. Specifically, patients with SLE manifested an increased 16 alpha hydroxylation of estradiol leading to compounds with significant peripheral estrogen potency. Indeed, a similiar finding of elevated 16 alpha hydroxyesterone was seen in male patients with SLE; in the females, however, elevations were noted in both 16 alpha hydroxyesterone and estriol [118–121].

This increased estrogenic activity has been linked by other investigators to abnormalities of suppressor cell function and increased autoantibody production. A good deal of work has been done in this area, as noted above, in the NZB/NZW F1 mouse model, in which androgens suppress and estrogens accelerate the lupus-like disease process. Further support for these theories is the finding that patients with Klinefelter's syndrome, an XXY condition, are predisposed to SLE and exhibit abnormal estrogen metabolism [118, 119, 122]. It seems quite clear that the immunoendocrine interaction among estrogen, androgen and immunocompetent cells and their environment play a role in Systemic Lupus Erythematosis [123–125].

Diseases of the central nervous system also have been linked with estrogen. In the Sprague-Dawley rat, experimental allergic encephalomyelitis can be modified by the administration of oral contraceptives containing estrogen and progesterone. In the short-term model, the oral contraceptives inhibited experimental allergic encephalomyelitis, in all likelihood related to the estrogenic moiety in the contraceptive preparations [127]. A clinical correlate of these findings can be seen in patients with multiple sclerosis in which exacerbations of disease are more infrequent during the latter months of pregnancy, at a time of high estrogen concentration. Furthermore, attacks of severe illness have been reported to be particularly common in the postpartum period, at a time when blood estrogen concentrations decrease precipitously [128–130].

Another immunologic disorder, hereditary angioedema, can be modified by the therapeutic use of exogenous hormones [131]. Hereditary angioedema is characterized by an abnormal C-1 esterase inhibitor related to either abnormally low serum concentrations of the material or to an abnormal protein. Although the disease is prevalent in equal numbers in both males and females, some woman feel that attacks increase during times of high estrogen stimulation. In a double blind controlled study, treatment with the androgenic agent, danazol, markedly decreased attacks of hereditary angioedema in the therapy group compared to the placebo group. This strikingly effective therapeutic trial was accompanied by a return to normal of C-2, C-4, and C-1 esterase inhibitor. Therefore, this disorder characterized by an inherited protein abnormality could be completely corrected biochemically in many patients by treatment with an anabolic, androgenic steroid. It is unknown whether this is related to an immunologic effect of the androgenic steroid, or to increased production of C-1 esterase inhibitor in the liver, related to the anabolic effects of danazol [131, 132].

Estrogen has also been implicated in differences in severity, expresssion of symptoms, and ultimate outcome in a variety of infectious disease processes [133–148]. Historically, diseases usually associated with a cellular immune response have been specifically noted to have differences in clinical manifestations and increased mortality in women, particularly during times of high serum estrogen concentrations.

Over the years, Asian influenza has been linked with deaths in women of childbearing age, particularly during pregnancy [137]. For the most part, these deaths were due to severe necrotizing pneumonia, which may or may not have been caused by the virus itself. This was specifically noted during the influenza years of 1957 and 1958 in Minnesota. During this period, there were 57 deaths from all causes associated with pregnancy, with influenza accounting for more deaths than any other cause, or 19.2% of the total. Obviously, these deaths may have been related to causes other than viral pneumonia, such as bacterial superinfection, decreased pulmonary function related to the mechanics of pregnancy, or perhaps other underlying diseases, such as mitral stenosis. However, in the Minnesota study, influenza A was cultured from the lung in three of the four patients in whom it was attempted [131)]. In addition, other reports from New Yorks City [149)] and England [150)] have noted an increased mortality rate during pregnancy related to Asian influenza. Therefore, although no indisputable conclusions can be drawn, there does appear to be an association between maternal influenza and periods of estrogenic hormonal stimulation.

In coccidioidomycosis, there is also a difference in immunologic phenomena related to the disease between men and women. Specifically, erythema nodosum is more commonly seen in women than in men. In a retrospective study of 432 residents. of the San Joaquin Valley who had experienced valley fever, only four men for every ten women were seen with this manifestation of disease. This is particularly fascinating when one considers that the incidence of dissemination of coccidioidomycosis is reversed compared to erythema nodosum with approximately four to seven men for every one woman involved. It should also be noted that the female predisposition to erythema nodosum does not occur before puberty [135)].

Most remarkable, however, is the effect of pregnancy, with its concommitant increased serum estrogen concentrations, on the outcome of primary benign coccidioidomycosis [133, 135, 138)]. Smale and Waechter [138)] report on 15 cases of coccidioidomycosis in pregnant women and indicate that the risk of death in these women is nearly 100% in untreated cases, and postulate that in indemic areas, it may be the leading cause of maternal deaths. Treatment with Amphotericin B may improve this prognosis. Other authors have also reported similar findings, with an increased incidence of fetal abnormalities as well. Whether the poor prognosis of coccidioidomycosis associated with pregnancy is related to the high serum estrogen concentrations and its effect on immune function is not clear, but further investigative work has been carried out regarding the effects of sex hormones on the causative organism, *Coccidioides immitis*. Drutz et al. [134)], have shown that, in vitro, estrogen accelerates the rate of spherule maturation and endospore release in a dose dependent fashion. In similar studies with *Cryptococcus neoformans*, Candida species, and *Petrollidium boydii* it was reported that growth was unaffected by the same concentrations of estradiol that had distinct effects on *C. immitis*. Mechanistically, *C. immitis* has been shown to have specific estrogen receptors and perhaps this may account for the increased in vitro growth in the presence of estrogen and for the pregnancy-related predisposition to dissemination and death related to this disease.

Estrogen has also been shown to affect macrophage Fc(IgG) receptor-mediated clearance of IgG coated erythrocytes at serum concentrations normally achieved during pregnancy in guinea pigs [151)]. Furthermore, estradiol at pharmacologic levels approximating those measured during pregnancy has been reported to inhibit neutrophil generation of superoxide anions as well as degranulation [152)]. This effect on superoxide anion production was maintained when 17 B estradiol was combined with progesterone in concentrations designed to approximate those seen in pregnancy. Specifically, estradiol inhibited beta glucuronidase and lysozyme release. Neutrophils isolated from women during various phases of the menstrual cycle and during the third trimester of pregnancy did not differ with respect to chemotactic peptide stimulated superoxide anion generation, suggesting that the inhibition of neutrophil responsiveness required adequate concentrations of the hormone to be maintained in the reaction mixure [152)]. This abnormality of leukocyte function may play a role in the incidence of death related to superinfection secondary to influenza as well as fungal diseases.

6 Effects of Androgens on Immune Responses

The androgens testosterone, 5-α-androstone-3,17-dione and dihydrotestosterone have all been reported to affect immune response [8-11, 76-79, 124, 153-155)]. For example, female hamsters posses a more active primary and secondary immune response than do males [67, 68, 156)], and this depression in the male hamster takes place shortly after sexual maturity when testosterone levels are increasing [156)]. In androgen-sensitive strains of female mice, treatment with testosterone results in a massive lymphocytosis, while in male mice of the same strain, testosterone treatment produces lymphophenia [154)]. Furthermore, in these mice, the males have lower titers of circulating IgM and IgG_2 than do females [124, 153)].

Treatment of chick embryos with testosterone has been reported to suppress the development of bursal follicles and produces hormonal bursectomy in chicks. As a result of this androgenization incomplete maturation of B-lymphocytes takes place, response to antigen is limited, and only IgM, but no IgG, is produced [157-161)]. Testosterone treatment also significantly reduces thymocyte numbers, possibly by interfering with the initial migration of bursal stem cells to the thymus [159)]. Furthermore, regeneration of thymus-independent areas of peripheral lymphoid tissues (composed mainly of B-lymphocytes) is inhibited by testosterone treatment, suggesting that testosterone acts on the differentiation of stem cells towards the population of bone marrow-derived B-lymphocytes [162-164)].

Mice and rats are also affected by the steroid 5-α-androstone-3,17-dione which depresses graft-vs.-host reactivity in spleen cells [155)], while dihydrotestosterone (DHT) (the 5α reduced metabolite of testosterone) has been reported to regulate the release of a serum factor that depresses PHA-stimulated blast transformation in vitro [8-11)]. DHT has also been shown to alter the course of murine lupus present in F_1 NZB/NZW mice. Females of this inbred strain normally develop this autoimmune disease and die, while the male is not as susceptible. However, female NZB/NZW mice will survive if treated with DHT, and males will die of this disease if castrated prepubertally [76-79, 125, 165)]. Furthermore, NZB and NZB hybrid male mice generate less antibody to T-cells and to single stranded DNA than do females, and this dimorphism is abolished by castration in the male and exacerbated in castrated females receiving testosterone implants [123, 166)]. Support for the hypothesis that suppressor T-cells function abnormally in the NZB animal is supplied by the observation that this animal model fails to develop tolerance to high levels of deaggregated bovine gammaglobulin [167)], but tolerance can be restored by treatment with testosterone. Furthermore, NZB strain animals possess T-cells, B-cells, and macrophages which all function abnormally, suggesting a lesion at the level of the stem cell [168)].

In humans, as in the NZB strain mouse, similar immunological alterations have been observed both clinically and experimentally. For example, systemic lupus erythematosis (SLE) is predominantly found in females and commonly takes the form of a heightened humoral and depressed cellular immunity [169)], combined with impairment of suppressor-cell function [119,122,170,171)]. Furthermore, in human SLE, as in the mouse model, androgen treatment suppresses and estrogen treatment accelerates these immunological abnormalities [119,122,170,171)]. These estrogen effects are especially pertinent considering that many SLE patients demonstrate alterations in steroid metabolism resulting in elevated levels of 16α-hydroxylated estrogen metabolites which can act as potent estrogens [120,121)].

SLE is not the only sex-related autoimmune disorder in humans. Rheumatoid arthritis is more prevalent in females than males, and the arthritic inflammation is significantly reduced in women using oral contraceptives [172–175)], suggesting that estrogens and progestins can modify the course of this disease. Estrogen treatment and castration have also been reported to increase the levels of circulating autoantibody in male mice suffering from experimental autoimmune thyroiditis, while testosterone treatment decreases autoantibody titers [176)].

Furthermore, experimental demyelinating disease in female rats appears to be inhibited by the estrogenic component of oral contraceptives [127)], while oral contraceptives are also known to depress various parameters of the cell-mediated immune response in women [177,178)].

In humans, the autoimmune-like disorder, idiopathic thrombocytopenic purpura (ITP) is more prevalent in women then in men. Symptoms of this disorder are exacerbated during menstruation, probably as a result of the decreasing levels of sex steroids at this time during the cycle, while androgen treatment has been reported to normalize platelet counts and reduce platelet reactive IgG [179,180)].

Sex differences are also noted in patients with Hepatitis B virus infection. Specifically, the incidence of the carrier state is greater in males post-HBsAg infection, as is the prevalence of chronic liver disease associated with this virus. Further evidence to substantiate these findings is seen when diseases associated with the Hepatitis B surface antigen are evaluated for differences in predisposition by sex. Chronic hepatitis, post-necrotic cirrhosis, primary hepatocellular carcinoma, Down's syndrome, chronic renal disease treated with hemodialysis, Hodgkin's disease, lepromatous leprosy, and polyarteritis nododosa, all are diseases in which the frequency of HBsAg carriers is higher than in the general population, and in which the disease has a higher prevalence among males than females. For some of these disorders, Hepatitis B virus is related to the etiology and/or pathogenesis of the disease, but for others, the carrier state may be related to abnormalities of the immune system, increasing the susceptibility to chronicity of the Hepatitis virus [140,141)].

It has been postulated that there is an antigen on the Hepatitis B virus that cross-reacts with a male-associated antigen in humans. This has been related to impaired graft survival in patients who are chronic carriers of HBsAg receiving post-renal transplantation grafts from male donors [181)]. It is tantalizing to postulate that the production of Hepatitis B surface antibody may cross-react with male-associated antigen on the donor kidney. Obviously, a good deal more work will be necessary before these theories can be substantiated.

Several other diseases have been associated with androgens in humans. Androgens have been related to insulin resistance and elevated fasting immunoreactive insulin in patients with polycystic ovary syndrome and although this may be related, in part, to obesity, the hyperinsulinemia has been correlated with testosterone and luteinizing hormone serum concentrations [182)]. In addition, Shoupe and Lobo [183)] have shown a positive serum correlation between testosterone and immunoreactive insulin, while there was a negative correlation with serum sex hormone binding globulin, in patients with idiopathic hirsutism. It is unclear whether this is immunologic in origin or secondary to feedback mechanisms relating hyperinsulinemia, increased serum testosterone, and the pituitary-hypophyseal axis. In the spontaneously diabetic BB rat, however, there is a profound immune defect relating to peripheral blood T-cells and pancreatic lymphocytic infiltration [184, 185)].

Neoplastic diseases have also been associated with androgen receptors in tumor tissue. Peliosis hepatis, hepatic tumors, both benign and malignant, and angiosarcomas have been linked to administration of exogenous androgens in patients with primary hematologic disorders, such as aplastic anemia. It is not known whether this tumorogenesis is related to the cytosolic hormone receptors known to exist in certain of these neoplasia or to some other unknown predisposition to secondary tumor formation [186)].

Testosterone receptors are present in prostatic tumors, and therapy for this disease is related to modulation of the hormonal environment of the individual. These hormonal manipulations may include castration and/or diethylstilbesterol therapy [187)].

Finally, alcoholic hepatitis, with perhaps transformation to hepatic fibrosis and cirrhosis, may be linked to an autoimmune phenomenon related to ethanol injured hepatocyte membrane or the degenerative scleral protein, the mallory body. A recent study has shown an encouraging therapeutic effect of the androgenic steroid, oxandrolone, in the therapy of this severe disease. It is not known whether this therapeutic success was due to the stimulation of protein synthesis by the androgenic steroid, or to changes in the immunocompetence of the host related to androgen therapy [188)].

7 Effects of Progesterone on Immune Response

Progesterone has also been reported to act as a potent inhibitor of the cell-mediated immune response. Skin graft survival is increased in hamsters, rats, mice, and monkeys treated with progesterone [189, 190)], while, in monkeys, progesterone treatment leads to lymphocytosis [190)]. Progesterone can also suppress spleen cell function in vivo and in vitro [190)], inhibit phytohemagglutinin-induced lymphocyte transformation and clonal formation [191, 192)] and generate significantly increased suppressor cell activity [193)]. Of interest is the observation that cyproterone acetate, an anti-androgen compound, has also been reported to retard skin graft rejection, to reduce the synthesis of antibody to sheep red blood cells and to damage lymphoid and thymic tissue [194)]. Theoretically, it might be expected that an anti-androgen like cyproterone should stimulate immune response, however, since cyproterone also possesses marked progestational activity, this could account for its immunoinhibitory properties [195)].

8 Effects of Gonadal Steroids on Immune Response During Pregnancy

During pregnancy, the immune response to a variety of agents is significantly depressed. As a result, the maternal-fetal rejection response is inhibited and pregnancy is maintained until term. On the other hand, in habitual aborters, this rejection response remains active [196)]. Support for a depression of the cell-mediated immune response during pregnancy can be found in a number of reports. For example, in pregnant women, cell-mediated immune response to rubella virus is depressed [197)], PHA [197–199)], and MLC responsiveness [197)] is decreased, tuberculin skin test (PPD) reactivity is inhibited [198, 200, 201)], and skin grafts survive longer without rejection [202)]. Further, in pseudo-pregnant rabbits, response to rubella virus is also decreased [203)], while in pregnant mice, contact sensitivity to picryl chloride is reduced [204)].

A variety of different factors have been proposed as immunoinhibitors during pregnancy. Steroids have been suggested since they are significantly elevated during this time. Progesterone, as well as 20α-dihydroprogesterone, has been shown to inhibit PHA-induced blastogenic transformation of lymphocytes [191, 192)], and the levels of steroid employed in these studies match those reported in human placenta [191, 192, 205)]. Progesterone in combination with estrone has also been shown to prolong skin graft survival in rats [206–208)], mice [209)], monkeys [210)] and hamsters [211)]. In humans, the levels of placental progesterone are in the range of 2×10^3—6×10^3 ng/g tissue [212–214)], and at those levels progesterone has been demonstrated to act as an immunosuppressive agent in vitro [191, 192, 205, 213)], and in vivo [210, 213, 215–218)].

Serum factors other than the progestens may also play a role in pregnancy-related immunosuppression, including maternal macrophage inhibitory factor, IgG antibody, estradiol, and cortisol. Another possible mechanism that has been suggested to account for the failure of rejection of the fetus is the presence of barriers that immunologically separate the placental and fetal tissue. Although this explanation may be partially correct, it would be simplistic to assume that this is the sole explanation for survival of the fetal allograft.

There is accumulating evidence, however, of specific immunosuppression during pregnancy, particularly in the latter stages. Specifically, during the second and third trimesters, maternal lymphocytes reveal a diminished proliferative response to soluble antigens, as well as allogeneic lymphocytes. Cell-mediated cytotoxicity, as reflected in killing of viral-infected cells, is also decreased during pregnancy. In addition, there is a decrease in numbers of T-helper/inducer lymphocytes during pregnancy [142, 219, 220)]

The thymus, which has much to do with regulation and maturation of T-lymphocytes, is significantly involuted and atrophied during pregnancy, and these changes include a reduction in cortical thymocytes, while medullary thymocytes remain unchanged [41–43)]. Cortical thymocytes have been reported to be glucocorticoid sensitive and are increased by steroid withdrawal after castration, while medullary thymocytes appear to be steroid resistant [40)]. Furthermore, medullary thymocytes demonstrate a greatly reduced response to both PHA and Con A [41)], which may explain, in part, the reduced immune response at this time.

Despite the occurrence of these various phenomenae, they only represent circumstantial evidence relating maternal immunosuppression to fetal allograft survival.

Adding to the case for clinical implications for this maternal immunosuppression are the variety of diseases which are increased during pregnancy. These include smallpox, polio, viral hepatitis, varicella-zoster, influenza, cytomegalovirus, and pulmonary and systemic mycoses [133–135, 137, 138, 142].

Although it is not possible to conclude that all of these events are related, it does appear that the immunosuppression associated with pregnancy has clinical significance, particularly in the area of infectious diseases and perhaps fetal allograft survival. This immunosuppression is, in all likelihood, multifactorial, and related both to steroid hormone production during pregnancy, as well as abberrations of lymphocyte activity, and changes in lymphocyte phenotypic subpopulations.

9 Regulation of the Immune Response by Adrenal Hormones

Glucocorticoids produced by the adrenal cortex have been well documented to depress immune responses. For example, the mitogenic response of lymphocytes in the presence of lectins is, in some instances, reduced by addition of glucocorticoids [212, 218, 221–223] but this response in vitro is variable and depends principally on the mitogen concentration used to stimulate blastogenesis [223].

One potent glucocorticoid which has been shown to alter in vitro colony growth is hydrocortisone. At high concentrations, hydrocortisone has variable effects on colony growth of myelogenous human leukemic cells, reducing in vitro growth of these cells from some patients but not from others [224]. On the other hand, hydrocortisone has been reported to exert a dose related reduction in colony formation of normal human T-lymphocytes which is abrogated with interlukin 2 (IL-2) treatment [225]. Also of interest is the study by Galanaud et al. [226], which demonstrated that hydrocortisone depression of a specific plaque forming cell response is dependent on the presence of monocytes in the culture. This is in agreement with an earlier study which showed that glucocorticoid depresssion of in vitro blast transformation requires monocytes to be present [223]. Furthermore, according to studies by Ambrose [227], corticosterones are required for in vitro induction of the immune response, and are also able to facilitate derepression of genes by unmasking sites on the DNA of chromatin for attachment of natural inducers [227].

The mechanism by which hydrocortisone can exert its effects on lymphocyte function may be related to its ability to alter membrane markers on the surface of those cells. In a study by Dupont, et al. [228], hydrocortisone induced a redistribution of the markers for immunoglobin Fc (Tm) receptors and T_4 receptors on the surface of helper lymphocytes. These findings may explain in part the immunosuppressive ability of glucocorticoids in human transplantation, and the observation that in well-tolerated transplants, suppressor cells are present [229–231]. It is possible that the cellular effects of hydrocortisone are mediated through cytoplasmic glucocorticoid receptors which have been reported to be present in lymphocytes [33–36, 38, 39, 232] since translocation of the steroid receptor complex into the nucleus can alter protein synthesis which might hypothetically affect structures present on the cell membrane surface.

Support for a link between glucocorticoid receptor binding and enzyme regulation of metabolism can be found in studies on cholesterol biosynthesis in isolated mouse thymocytes [233]. In this model system, dexamethasone has been shown to produce a marked inhibition of cholesterol biosynthesis and this inhibitory effect is specific for glucocorticoids and not other steroids, suggesting receptor binding is involved. Furthermore, this decrease in cholesterol synthesis produced by dexamethasone is abolished in the presence of Actinomycin D, implying that these effects are mediated via glucocorticoid receptor occupancy and macromolecular protein synthesis [233]. Treatment with glucocorticoids has been reported to either delay graft rejection responses [234-236], have no effect on graft rejection responses [237-239], or stimulate graft rejection responses [240], depending on the animal model, technique, or concentration of glucocorticoid utilized. Furthermore, glucocorticoids have also been shown to depress antibody production [241-249], inhibit T-cell (250, 251) and NK effector cell [252,253] function and depress the inflammatory response capacity of macrophages [254]. Injection of rats or rabbits with cortisone was also able to reduce the number of small lymphocytes in thymus independent areas, produce thymic cortical atrophy, germinal center atrophy and arrest the migration of B-lymphocytes from the bone marrow to the germinal centers in the peripheral lymphoid organs [255]. Treatment with the potent glucocorticoid, prednisolone, resulted first in an increased release of small lymphocytes from the thymus, followed later by a marked decrease in lymphocyte release [256]. These studies suggest that glucocorticoids function to modulate lymphocyte responsiveness as well as regulate transport of these cells between immunological compartments.

Alterations in the hormonal environment in vivo by organ ablation have also been reported to affect the immune response. For example, serum prepared from adrenalectomized rats was significantly more stimulatory in blastogenic assay on intact thymic cells than was serum from control animals [7]. While castrate serum has also been shown to stimulate suppressor T-lymphocyte blast transformation in vivo, the serum prepared from combined castrate-adrenalectomized rats was significantly more stimulatory than serum for either single ablation animal [7]. Furthermore, in animals thymectomized, hypophysectomized and treated with thymic hormone, it was reported that circulating thymic hormone was a synergist to circulating hypophyseal growth hormone, and an antagonist to circulating corticotropin [240]. This finding may have a bearing on immunological regulation by the hypothalamic-pituitary-adrenal-thymic (HPAT) axis since glucocorticoids are thought to play a role in regulation of factors released by the thymus (see below). Other factors which are known to affect response of immunocompetent cells, and which are also under the control of glucorticoids, are interleukins 1 and 2. In three separate studies, it was reported that glucocorticoids inhibited the production and/or action of these interleukins [257-259], suggesting an additional mechanism by which glucocorticoids could depress immune response.

Recently, Besedovsky, et al.[260] reported that blood lymphocytes in culture produced a glucocorticoid-increasing factor (GIF) which significantly elevated corticosterone in rats [260]. Of special interest was the observation that GIF functioned directly at the level of the pituitary and not at the adrenal glands (possibly by regulating ACTH release), since hypophysectomy inhibited the GIF response. These findings imply that a lymphocyte-mediated immunoregulatory mechanism exists that is apparently separate from the feedback pathways which alter release of thymic hormones.

Stress is another factor that can alter circulating levels of glucocorticoid as well as inhibit immune response. For example, in patients with major depression, significantly elevated levels of corticoreleasing factors have been reported [261], while in lymphocytes obtained from spouses bereaved after the death of their mates, there was a significant depression in both PHA and Con A responsiveness, although the levels of circulating cortisol in these subjects were similar to controls [262].

In major thermal burn patients, a good correlation has been found between anergy to skin tests performed in vivo and serum suppression of PHA lymphocyte response in vitro, but this anergy does not appear to be correlated with serum cortisol levels [263]. Stress due to protein malnutrition also appears to alter the immune response. In mice fed a low (0–4%) protein diet, lymphocyte PHA and LPS responsiveness was depressed, while corticosterone levels were elevated. These abnormalities could, to some degree, be corrected by treatment with thymosin fraction 5 [264], suggesting that the Hypothalamic-Pituitary-Adrenal-Thymic (HPAT) axis might, in some way, be involved in stress-related immune depression.

Stress in aged male rats also appears to increase their vulnerability to various pathological disorders. According to a study by Sapolsky and Donelly [265], because aged male rats show a delay in terminating corticosterone secretion after the abatement of stress, they are more susceptible to stress-induced tumor growth. Furthermore, stimulation of this aged pattern of corticosterone hypersecretion in young animals using steroid administration can also generate an increase in tumor growth [265]. Such hyperadrenocorticism in aging is also thought to contribute to atherosclerosis, osteoporosis and steroid diabetes [266].

Immunity to bacterial and viral infections also has been reported to be reduced by glucocorticoids. For example, in animals compromised by elevated levels of glucocorticoids, experimentally-induced *Klebsiella pneumoniae* infection spreads more rapidly than in controls [267], while host defenses to intracellular pathogens are depressed by cortisol treatment [268] and sera from cortisol-treated mice possesses reduced anti-viral activity with respect to serum from non-cortisol-treated animals [269].

A wide variety of corticosteroid preparations are used in clinical medicine for the primary purpose of suppressing inflammation. Whenever the inflammatory response may be detrimental to the host, corticosteroids are employed to ameliorate the unwanted inflammatory activity. Specifically, corticosteroids delay and diminish DNA synthesis in lymphocytes, decrease production of lymphokines, change lymphocyte subset pools, and diminish lymphocyte proliferative responses [270–270]. Corticosteroids also impact the granulocytic series of inflammatory cells by decreasing adherence and subsequent margination and diapedesis, and perhaps impairing production of soluble mediators of inflammation [276, 277]. These effects are dramatic, and have both positive and negative implications in the therapy of human disease.

Corticosteroids have been positively employed in the treatment of infectious diseases such as retinochoriditis and unveitis related to *Toxiplasma gondii* and facial herpetic disease, in which the inflammatory response can lead to worsened visual acuity and post-herpetic neuralgia, respectively. There is some evidence that corticosteroid therapy may be beneficial in cases of septic shock, perhaps related to stabilization of lysosomal membranes and decreased degranulation of polymorphonuclear leukocytes. It has also been suggested that cortiosteroids may inhibit endorphin activity associated with the vasodilatation seen in septic shock although further proof is required [276]. Corticosteroids are also used extensively in other immunologic disorders, such as systemic lupus erythematosis, myasthenia gravis, organ transplantation, and a variety of lymphoproliferative hematologic malignancies [122, 278, 279].

Use of corticosteroids in any of these settings can be associated with adverse effects as well. Specifically, there is an increase in incidence of superinfection in patients treated with long-term corticosteroid therapy [278]. This is, in all likelihood, related to the impaired immune response in individuals so treated. The organisms that are most commonly seen in patients with long-term corticosteroid therapy are those that have been related to the cellular-immune response in humans, such as the systemic mycoses, viral diseases, and certain parasitic diseases such as *Pneumocystis carinii* pneumonia. Although a great deal more work is necessary in order to relate the therapeutic effects of corticosteroids with the basic pathobiology of immunologic diseases, it seems clear that these compounds dramatically impair immune function. Such impairment may act either positively producing beneficial results or have a negative impact depending on the clinical setting.

10 Regulation of the Immune Response by Pituitary Hormones

10.1 Effects of Hypophysectomy

Since the pituitary is known to play a major role in regulation of other endocrine organs, it is not surprising to find that removal of the pituitary results in alterations in immune response. In a series of studies by Nagy and Berczi, hypophysectomy in rats has been reported to depress both contact dermatitis, rejection of skin grafts, and antibody production, and these effects could be reversed to varying degrees, either by normal pituitary or pituitary tumor transplants, or by replacement hormonal therapy utilizing prolactin, somatotropin (growth hormone) or placental lactogen [280–285].

Hypophysectomy has also generated information relating to the neuroimmunomodulation of the pituitary gland. According to a study by Cross, et al. [286], lesions in the hypothalamus produce thymic involution and decrease splenocyte blastogenic responses, while lesions in the limbic areas increase thymic and splenic cellularity and stimulate mitogenic responses. Furthermore, hypophysectomy abrogates all of these changes produced by lesions in the hypothalamus and limbic systems. The results strongly support the hypothesis that neuroimmunomodulation is mediated predominantly by the pituitary [286].

Pituitary function also appears to be an integral factor in regulation of immunological responsiveness of aged animals. In many reports, the immunological responsiveness which declines with age was shown to be significantly restored by hypophysectomy [287–289]. For example, middle-aged rats receiving endocrine supplementation with a mixture of corticosterone, deoxycorticosterone and thyroxin were able to reject xenografts, clear carbon and produce antibodies significantly better after hypophysectomy [288, 290–292]. Denckla [293] has proposed that hypophysectomy prevents the age related decline in tissue responsiveness to thyroxin. This suggests that the pituitary releases a factor that decreases the ability of lymphocytes to respond to thyroxin [288], but other pituitary hormones may also be of importance in immune response.

10.2 *Effects of Somatotropin*

Somatotropin (or growth hormone) has been reported to effectively stimulate immune response, both in vivo and in vitro. In in vivo studies, animals hypophysectomized for 15 weeks showed a significant drop in plaque-forming cells, hemagglutinin titers and DNA synthesis in lymphoid organs. When bovine growth hormone was administered to these hypophysectomized animals, there was an enhancement of lymphoid cell DNA synthesis and recovery of the immune response [294, 295]. Furthermore, somatotropin not only increased incorporation of thymidine-^{3}H into DNA^{35} in thymic cortical cells, but also incorporation of sodium sulfate-^{35}S into biopolymers produced in the thymic medulla [294, 295] and these effects were reversed by injection of anti-growth hormone antibody into the animals [294, 295]. Spleen cells transplanted from a donor to in vitro cultures have also been reported to be affected by hypophysectomy. Cells removed from hypophysectomized, but not adrenalectomized, donors were less antigen responsive than cells from normal donors. If, however, the hypophysectomized donor was treated with somatotropin prior to cell culture the cells reacted normally in culture when exposed to antigen [296]. Production of precipitating antibody in rats as measured by the hemagglutination and immunodiffusion tests is also depressed in hypophysectomized and thymectomized animals. While antibody production in this model could not be restored with either growth hormone or thymic hormone alone, it was restored when both these hormones were injected together [297], suggesting that a synergistic relationship may exist [240]. Furthermore, in a study by Arrenbrecht and Sorkin [298], it was reported that growth hormone was able to enhance helper function of normal thymocytes but not of lymph node cells, spleen cells or hydrocortisone-resistant thymocytes. Since cortisone-resistant thymocytes have been identified in the thymic medulla [40], and are also reduced during pregnancy [41], this implies that the growth hormone sensitive cells are located in the thymic cortex. Also of interest was a report by Pierpaoli and Sorkin [299], in which an antiserum raised against mouse pituitary acidophils also bound to and agglutinated thymocytes due to cross reacting antibody [299]. Pituitary acidophils are the cells which synthesize and release growth hormone, suggesting a similarity in surface antigen on both types of cells.

Growth hormone appears to produce more than one effect on lymphocytes. As has been reported by Arrenbrecht and Sorkin, it can enhance helper function [298], however, in a study by Snow, et al. [300], in vitro growth hormone allowed for the generation of cytotoxic T lymphocytes. Other studies support this stimulatory response seen in vitro, either in the presence of the mitogen, PHA, [301–303] or without mitogen [304], although one study found no effect [305]. A report by Grossman and Roselle [8] also demonstrated that growth hormone acting in vitro at a physiological concentration of 40 μg/ml could produce a depression in blastogenic transformation in the presence of either the mitogens PHA or Con A if rat serum was also added to the assay wells. These results suggest that a serum factor involved in lymphocyte regulation may be present.

The fact that growth hormone has been shown in many studies to stimulate the formation of immunocompetent thymocytes [298, 301–304, 306] is of interest when one considers runt disease. This disorder can be produced by infusing immature immunoincompetent donor thymocytes into young recipient animals. In classical runt disease as described by Billingham [307], epidermal erythema, exfoliation and dermatitis are present, growth is arrested, splenomegaly is usually apparent, and lymphoblasts and lymphocytes are absent in the lymphatic tissue [307]. These changes which produce runt diseases are due to graft-vs-host reactions and can be exacerbated by treatment with growth hormone, apparently, because growth hormone induces maturation of immunoincompetent donor thymocytes in the recipient into immunocompetent T-cells [306].

While runt disease can be attributed to overactivity of mature T-cells, when lymphocytes are unable to mature we have what is commonly referred to as wasting disease. Also studied by Pierpaoli and Sorkin [299, 308], this disorder can be induced by neonatal thymectomy, resulting in a decrease in growth rate, a decrease in peripheral blood leukocytes and depressed immune response. Similar results can also be produced by treating animals with either anti-thymus, anti-pituitary serum, or anti-somatotropic serum [299, 308], suggesting an interaction between these two organs regulated by growth hormone. Such an interaction is also supported by the fact that neonatal thymectomy produced changes in the acidophilic pituitary cells that produce growth hormone [308]. Since the effects of this wasting syndrome can be alleviated by treatment with growth hormone, this suggests that in young animals a deficiency in somatotropic hormone inhibits thymus mitotic activity. Such hormone-dependent mitotic activity could be essential in the thymus of young animals for a normal development of the immune system [308].

Support for this hypothesis can be found in studies with either dwarf mice or dwarf dogs. In the Snell-Bagg hypopituitary dwarf mouse, the levels of growth hormone are far below normal circulating concentrations [306], thymocytes are depleted from the thymic cortex [309], the levels of T and B lymphocytes are half the value found in normal litter mates [310], dwarf mice demonstrate a depression of both the humoral and cell mediated primary immune response [311–313], and die within 45–150 days after birth [306]. When dwarf mice are treated with either growth hormone alone or growth hormone and thyroxin, the hypotrophic thymus and lymph nodes can be reconstituted, immune responsiveness is normalized and the animals live for a year or more [306, 311, 313].

Dwarf Weimaroner dogs, like Snell-Bagg mice, are also susceptible to wasting disease. These inbred dogs have small thymus glands with a marked absence of thymic cortex, a depressed lymphocyte blast response to mitogens, and plasma growth hormone levels which do not increase after an injection of clonidine HCl as they do in normal litter mates [314, 315]. Treatment with either growth hormone or thymosin fraction five produces clinical improvement in these animals [314, 315].

Since the absence of growth hormone is able to produce wasting syndrome in dwarf dogs and Snell/Bagg mice, it is of interest to ascertain if a similar clinical picture is present in humans. Unfortunately, the effects of growth hormone on the human immune response is at present equivocal. In studies by Thieriot-Prevost et al. [316], there was a clear relationship between the uptake of ^{3}H-thymidine into lectin-activated lymphocytes and the hormonal content of the patient serum such that serum from acromegalic patients was more stimulatory than serum from hypopituitary dwarfs. The authors hypothesize that this response may be due to variations in somatomedin levels [316)].

Support for these results can be found in preliminary work by Bajoruunas et al. [317)], who studied adults with active acromegaly, adults with hypopituitary growth hormone deficiency, and children with growth hormone deficiency. It was found that in many patients, abnormalities were present in the levels of circulating immunoglobins, while in growth hormone deficient children who had previously received therapy for hand and neck malignancies, lymphocyte mitogen or antigen responsiveness was depressed. These abnormalities were corrected by growth hormone replacement therapy [317)]. It has also been demonstrated that in some children with acute lymphoblastic leukemia, growth hormone and somatomedin levels are elevated and may be reduced after remission is achieved [318)]. This observation appears pertinent since in rats suffering from T-cell leukemia, hypophysectomy can suppress the leukemic process [318)], suggesting that the cancer is supported by somatotropin or other hormones elaborated by the pituitary.

On the other hand, neither Ammann, et al. [319)] nor Abbassi and Bellanti [320)] in their research were able to demonstrate a significant connection between growth hormone levels and immunological function in patients with growth hormone deficiency.

10.3 *Effects of Prolactin*

As has been previously discussed, in the hypophysectomized animal model, both humoral and cell-mediated immune responses are depressed, but replacement with prolactin reconstitutes the immune reactivity. For example, IgM and IgG antibody response to sheep red blood cells in hypophysectomized female rats could be restored by syngeneic pituitary grafts or by prolactin treatment [280, 281)], as could contact sensitivity to dinitrochlorobenzene [280, 282–284)]. In a preliminary study, it was also reported that the immunorestorative effect exerted by prolactin is dose-dependent and, further, that bromocriptine, a prolactin antagonist, decreased immunocompetence in normal rats [320)]. In support of the immunorestorative properties of prolactin is a study by Sotowska-Brochocka, et al. [321)], who demonstrated that in chickens, prolactin administration increased production of anti-sheep red blood cell antibody, as well as number of lymphocytes. Of interest is the finding that prolactin was able to induce expression of Thy-l antigen on 14-day fetal thymic stem cells in culture [322)], suggesting that prolactin can stimulate maturation of immature thymocytes into mature T-cells.

While prolactin in most reports acts to stimulate immune response, in a study carried out in vitro, it was shown that at elevated levels of prolactin (75 μg/ml), lymphocyte transformation was depressed, but this was not the case at normal physiological concentrations (15 μg/ml) [323)]. In this study, it was also reported that treatment of mice in vivo with the prolactin-suppressing drug bromoergokryptine reduced the weight of all organs except the thymus [323)].

Prolactin has also been implicated in the reconstitution of immune reactivity in the nude mouse model. In an elegant study by Pierpaoli, Kopp and Bianchi [324)], it was shown that immunological blockade of anteriopituitary function by anti-pituitary antibodies in thymic nude mice bearing skin grafts prevented reconstitution of transplant immunity when these animals received thymic grafts. On the other hand, thymic grafts in nude mice with functional anterior pituitary glands were found to reconstitute the immune response and accelerated skin graft rejection. In athymic nude mice, prolactin levels were also reported to be reduced, while luteotropic hormone levels were elevated and implantation of thymus normalized blood levels of the hormones [324]. These results support the hypothesis of a two-way interaction between thymus and pituitary and affirm the role of the thymus in organizing maturing brain for endocrine functions. They also support the view that prolactin is involved in early immunodifferentiation. Prolactin release from the pituitary also appears to be regulated by gonadal function since the nonaromatizable androgen, dihydrotestosterone, and the pure progestin, R5020, have been shown to act directly at the pituitary level to inhibit spontaneous prolactin release and also reduce the well known stimulatory effect of estradiol on prolactin release [325-327].

11 Effects of Thyroid Hormones

Among the growing list of hormones required to maintain proper immune reactivity are triiodothyronine (T_3) and thyroxin (T_4) which are produced by the thyroid gland. In the hypopituitary dwarf mouse model in order to completely reconstitute humoral and cell mediated immunity both thyroxin and somatotropin are necessary [311,313]. Support for the importance of thyroid hormone can be demonstrated when one considers the effect of treating mice with antibodies against thyroid hormone. As with anti-somatotropic antibody, anti-thyrotrophic antibody produced a marked thymic and lymphoid organ involution along with a depression in antibody production [311]. Similarly in rats infected with plerocercoid larvae of *Spirometra mansonoids* levels of both growth hormone and thyroxin spontaneously decreased by two weeks post infection and then returned to normal by 4 to 9 weeks [328]. During the period when hormone levels were reduced a suppression in immune response was also observed which normalized as hormonal concentration increased. If rats infected with plerocercoid larvae also received daily injections of either T_4 or growth hormone the immune response returned to normal in the T_4 injected animals but not in those treated with growth hormone [328].

Blockage of thyroxine release in mice and rats with propyl-thiouracil (PTU) also resulted in a depression of immune response. After 20 days of such treatment relative spleen weight was reduced while relative thymic weight was not changed by comparison with untreated controls. In these PTU animals the primary immune response to sheep red blood cells was also greatly impaired. Furthermore, a full reversal and recovery from these conditions could be obtained by injecting the PTU-treated animals with thyroxine [306].

Treatment of adult (64 week old) hypophysectomized rats with thyroxine has also been reported to shorten xenograft rejection time from 13.8 days to 6.5 days and accelerate carbon clearance by phagocytic cells [329]. Furthermore, suppressor (but not helper) T-lymphocytes are reduced in hypothyroid rats [330] and suppressor T-cells are increased upon treatment with triiodothyronine (T_3) [331].

Alteration in levels of circulating thyroid hormones due to an underlying immunological lesion, or conversly alterations in immune response as a result of changes in circulating thyroid hormones have been described in detail in extensive reviews on Graves and Hoshimoto's disease [332, 333]. In Graves disease circulating suppressor cells may be reduced, possibly due to the elevated levels of thyroxine [332]. Also in Graves disease, the TSH receptor may act as an antigen [334, 335] to generate antibodies which react with the TSH receptor to either block or stimulate cAMP and iodine uptake [333]. Antibody classes which have been reported to bind to TSH receptor include IgM, IgA, IgE with the majority identified as a heterogenous IgG population [333]. With respect to the underlying causes of Graves disease Burman and Baker suggest that it represents "a heterologous disorder with mutiple autoantibodies against multiple, different TSH binding sites" [333].

The hyperthyroidism of Graves disease surprisingly has many elements of similarity to the hypothyroidism of Hashimoto's disease. For example, in both disorders thyroid autoantibodies are present, the thyroid is infiltrated by lymphocytes, T-cells are sensitized to thyroid cell antigens and the hyperthyroidism present in Graves disease may spontaneously become the hypothyroidism of Hashimoto's disease or visa versa [332]. On the other hand, Kudd et al. [332]. points out that despite these close relationships, there are enough elements that separate Grave's from Hashimoto's disease, marking them as separate entities rather than merely extremes of a spectrum of a single entity.

12 Effect of Thymosins

Thymic hormones or thymosins are peptide hormones [44, 45] which have been reported to mediate development of various kinds of T-cell subsets (Fig. 5). Thymosin α_1 is hypothesized to stimulate stem cells to develop into prothrombocytes in the bone marrow and T-helper cell formation in lymphoid tissue [12], while thymosin α_7 stimulates suppressor T-cell formation in the lymphoid tissue [12]. In an attempt to identify the mechanism by which thymosin stimulates T-cell action Naylor et al. [48] has studied the effects of thymosin fraction 5 (a crude preparation) on murine thymocytes. Using radioimmunoassays to measure both adenosine 3′ 5′ cyclic monophosphate (cAMP) and guanosine 3′ 5′ cyclic monophosphate (cGMP) they reported that cGMP levels, but not cAMP levels were significantly elevated in murine thymocytes which had been incubated with thymosin fraction 5.

As we have discussed earlier in this chapter, the thymic reticuloendothelial cells contain steroid receptors [19–24], and it is these cells which are also thought to produce thymic hormones. Therefore, it is not surprising to discover that thymic function is intimately associated with the function of the reproductive system. For example, studies were performed in both mice and rats in which the thymus was removed neonatally and the effects on the ovaries were observed. In mice neontally thymectomized on day 3, ovarian dysgenesis was demonstrated after thymectomy as characterized by lymphocytic infiltration of follicles, a decline in oocyte numbers and hypertrophy

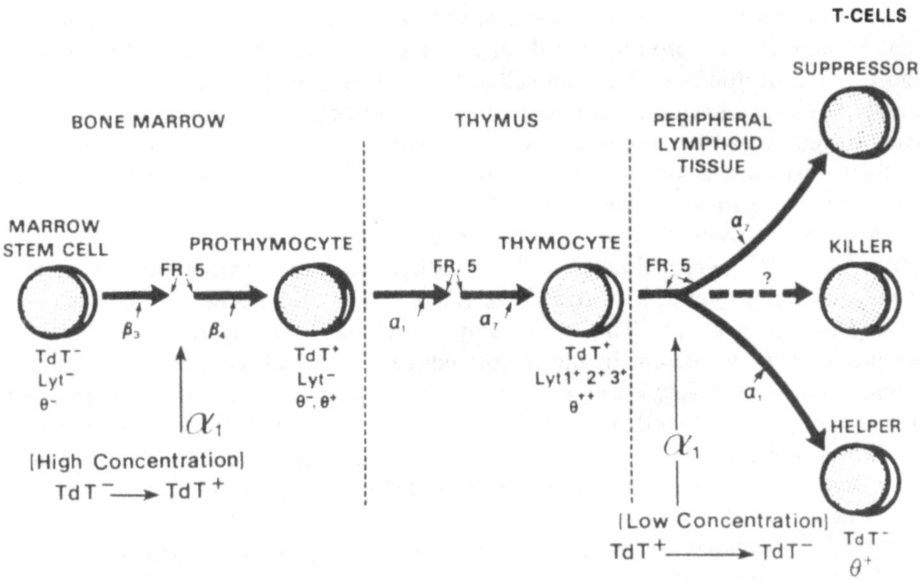

Fig. 5. Proposed role of thymosin peptids in T lymphocyte maturation. (Reprinted with permission from Low TLK, Thurman GB, Zata MM, Hu SK, Goldstein AL 1981 ADVANCES IN IMMUNOPHARMACOLOGY, Pergamon Press, England p. 71)

of the interstitial cellular elements [336–342]. Also in neonatally thymectomized male rats, testicular atrophy was present along with hypertrophy of pituitary B-cells, and thymectomy in female rats reduced progestins but not estrogen [341]. Other investigators have reported that in inbred strain mice thymectomized on day 3 after birth serum progesterone and estrogen were both reduced along with leutinizing hormone (LH), follicle stimulating hormone (FSH) and growth hormone, while thymosin levels were elevated [338–340]. The thymosin α_1 produced here is believed to originate from other organs, possibly by a mechanism of derepression, when the thymus is removed.

The mechanisms by which the thymus can affect the gonads both structurly and functionally is presently under investigation by a few groups of researchers located in various countries. Results seem to suggest that at least two separate but interrelated mechanisms are responsible. According to one hypothesis the maturity of the thymocyte accounts for thymic gonadal interaction. In the day 3 thymectomized animals helper T-cells are present but suppressor T-cells are absent having not matured before removal of the thymus. Thus, in the presence of helper T-cells, B-cells would produce autoantibodies against the oocytes [338, 342]. This theory, in effect, proposes that as a result of autoantibodies in the neonatally thymectomized animal young follicles are forced into early senescence. Such forced early senescence is supported by the theories of Bukovsky and Presl [343], Espey [344] and Farooki [345] who suggest that follicular atresia and regulation of ovulation and reproductive cycle result from immunological responses at the level of the ovary.

The second mechanism which may account for thymic-ovarian interactions is based on immunoendocrine axes and will be discussed at the end of this chapter.

The parathymic syndromes associated with abnormalities of the thymus gland are legion, and include neuromuscular disorders, such as myasthenia gravis; hematologic and protein disorders, such as red cell aplasia and autoimmune hemolytic anemia; endocrine disorders, such as thyrotoxicosis and thymic carcinoid; cutaneous disorders, such as mucocutaneous candidiasis; connective tissue diseases, such as systemic lupus erythematosis; and a wide variety of miscellaneous disorders, such as the myasthenic syndrome and giant cell myocarditis [278, 279, 346–354].

Perhaps the best-studied of these thymus-associated diseases is myasthenia gravis [278, 279, 351]. Approximately 15% of patients with myasthenia gravis have thymoma and salutory effects on relapse rates and remission have been seen in patients undergoing thymectomy. This effect may be related to removal of acetylcholine receptors normally present in the thymic epithelium, which could be antigenically similar to muscular acetylcholine receptors. Thus, thymectomy may both remove a reservoir of primed thymic lymphocytes, and, perhaps, eliminate a source of thymic hormones, which could impact on the systemic cellular immune function. This latter conclusion is attractive, although immunologic studies in patients post-thymectomy have shown varied results with no clear abberrations of immune function found, except for a decreased percentage of T-cells and a slightly increased primary immune response of lymphocytes.

The remainder of the disorders associated with abnormalities of thymic tissue have been less well studied. For example, thymectomy has been attempted in patients with systemic lupus erythamotosis with subsequent failure to improve the clinical sequelae of this disease [350]. This is in contrast to the beneficial effect of thymectomy in patients with myasthenia gravis [278, 351]. In patients with systemic lupus erythamotosis and thymoma, the major associated problem is an increased incidence of thymic malignancy, although no predominant histologic pattern has been observed [350].

Approximately 50% of patients with pure red-cell aplasia will have thymoma, and approximately 25–30% of that group will derive benefit from thymectomy [350]. The link between thymic abnormalities and pure red-cellaplasia is not clearly understood, but it must be noted that abnormalities of the thymus have also been related to a wide variety of malignant and non-malignant hematologic disorders.

13 Effects of Circadian Rhythm on Immune Response

In both rats and humans, various physiologic functions have been reported to be altered by variations in circadian rhythm. Glycolysis, oxidative metabolism and biliary functions are all maximum during the nocturnal activity phase [355–363]. Further, experimental results show that functional parameters of cell divison vary, depending on the time of observation during the light-dark cycle. The mitotic index of regenerating liver is maximal during the day and minimal during the night [364, 365] as in other tissues presenting either spontaneous or induced mitosis [355, 366]. Apparently, the passage from the G_0 (cells not engaged in cell division, but capable of differentiating) to G_1 (presynthesis) phase is influenced by circadian rhythm [363]. These observations are especially pertinent considering that clonal formation during the immune response depends on cell division (blastogenic transformation). This implies that variations in circadian rhythm could theoretically affect the development of precursor lymphocytes into adult, immunocompetent forms.

Length of day has also been shown to restrict reproductive behavior in a variety of animals. In rodents, exposure to short photoperiods results in involution of both the gonads and accessory glands [367, 368]. In rats in which testosterone [367] was neonatally administered, a marked increase in sensitivity to light deprivation was reported [360, 370]. Furthermore, short photoperiods were for more effective in reducing reproductive organ weights than longer photoperiods in neonatally treated animals [371].

In order to determine how these variations in photoperiod could alter reproductive weight, pinealectomies were performed. It was shown that pinealectomy prevented the decrease in reproductive organ weights induced by short photoperiods [371]. Since an increase in melatonin synthesis has been show to take place in the dark [372], it follows that short photoperiodic animals would be expected to posses longer lasting levels of melatonin than long photoperiodic animals. Longer lasting melatonin has indeed been reported in short photoperiodic animals along with an increase in activity of the enzyme N-acetyl-transferase, which is responsible for melatonin synthesis [371].

The relationship between photoperiod and reproductive organ weight appears to be mediated by the suppression of LH and FSH release from the pituitary by melatonin [373] via the Pineal Hypothalamic-Pituitary (PHP) axis. Since these gonadotropins regulate reproductive organ weight and function, it follows that short photoperiodic animals would be expected to have smaller reproductive organs and a decrease in circulating gonadal steroids.

Support for circadian rhythm in the immune response can be found in studies which demonstrate that in mice maximum immune reactivity (as measured by tumor development) is present during the dark phase while minimal immune reactivity is obtained during the light phase [374]. In sensitized animals, maximum oxazolone response can be obtained if the challenge occurs two hours before the onset of light [375], while murine plaque forming cell (PFC) response to sheep red blood cells (SRBC) is optimal if the animals are injected with SRBC near the onset of light [376]. Further, in Swiss Webster mice, an inverse relationship exists between peak thymosin α_1 levels and corticosterone [377]. In this mouse model (where the lights were on from 0700 to 1900 (7 a.m. to 7 p.m.) thymosin α_1 levels peak aroung 0800 (8 a.m.), while corticosterone levels reach a high at about 1700 (5 p.m.). This suggests that the circadian periodicity of serum thymosin α_1 is probably synchronized to the light-dark cycle [377]. Finally, a similar diurnal rhythm of thymosin α_1 is present in humans and is opposite to that of cortisol [378] such that cortisol levels are highest at 8 a.m. and lowest at 10 p.m. [378]. Collectively, these studies suggest that a relationship may exist between the pineal and the regulatory axes that govern the hypothalamus, pituitary, gonads and adrenals (see next section).

In animal models, the relationship between the pineal gland and the retina during the course of experimental autoimmune uveitis has also been studied [379]. In both guinea pigs and rats, it has been shown that when animals are immunized with S-antigen, with or without *Bordetella pertussis* adjuvant, mononuclear infiltrates occur both in the retina and in the pineal gland. In rats at least, this involvement is dependent upon the rat strain used with low responders for experimental autoimmune uveitis also developing a similar decrease in mononuclear cell infiltrate in the pineal gland after challenge with S-antigen. The implications of this finding with regard to the secretory functions of the pineal gland are, at this time, unclear.

14 Regulation of the Immune System by Hormonal Axes

14.1 The Hypothalamic-Pituitary Gonodal-Thymic (HPGT) Axis

From the previous discussion it is apparent that androgens, estrogens, progestins, glucocorticoids and some pituitary factors strongly influence the immune response. However, in a study by Williams et al. [380] it was reported that in female mice made immunodeficient by whole body irradiation the levels of both estradiol and progesterone decreased. Although the authors suggest that the cause of this decrease in both estrogen and progesterone could result from radiation damage to the ovaries, another explanation may exist. While it is clear that steroid hormones and pituitary factors are able to regulate thymic development and function [381] it is only just becoming apparent that thymic hormones can regulate pituitary function and subsequent release of LH. If irradiation limits thymic hormone release than the levels of LH would drop and gonadal function decrease. Thus, production of sex steroids from the gonads would be inhibited.

To elucidate possible humoral interactions between thymus and pituitary Rebar et al. [336, 337, 382] utilized a hypothalamic-pituitary perfusion system. With this in vitro model they were able to introduce thymic hormones into the chamber containing hypothalamic tissue and monitor production of releasing hormones by measuring the release of pituitary hormones from the chamber containing the hypophyseal tissue. They found that thymosin fraction 5 (a crude parent preparation containing thymosins α_1 and B_4) when introduced into the hypothalamic chamber stimulated the release of GnRH from the hypothalamus and LH release from the pituitary. Support for the ability of thymosin to release LH from the pituitary can be found in work with mice intravenously injected with thymosins [383]. In this model injection with thymosin B_4 significantly elevated serum LH levels, whereas injection with thymosin fraction 5 significantly decreased serum LH and injection with thymosin α_1 showed no change in serum LH.

Armed with the knowledge that thymosin B_4 stimulates LH release from the pituitary we can now explain why there is a reduced secretion of gonadotropins and testosterone in athymic mice [384, 385] and why early thymectomy in mice delays vaginal opening and reduces gonodotropin secretion [338–340, 386].

In addition to the effect of thymosin B_4 on gonadotropin release, thymosin α_1 levels have been reported to be reduced by in vivo estradiol treatment [387] implying that estradiol inhibits thymosin release. Thus we have demonstrated that the thymic-gonadal relationships depend on a series of interactive functions between the hypothalamus, pituitary, gonads and thymus, currently described as the HPGT axis.

According to this scheme the HPGT axis functions as follows (Fig. 6). Release of the thymic hormone, thymosin B_4, stimulates the hypothalamus to release gonadotropin releasing hormone (GnRH) which in turn release LH and FSH from the pitui-

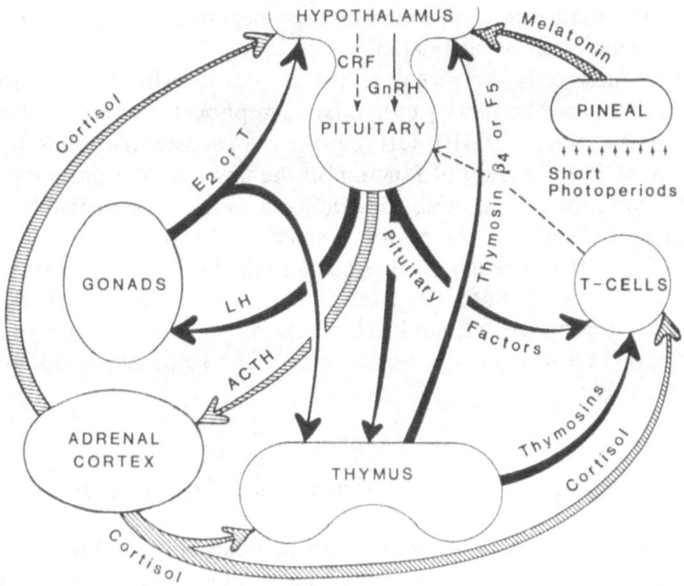

Fig. 6. Hypothetical scheme for the regulation of T lymphocytes by the HPGT axis, HPAT axis and PHP axis

tary. These gonadotropins then stimulate gonadal function and release of sex steroid hormones. Negative feedback of the sex steroids onto the hypothalamus-pituitary inhibits gonadotropin release and decreases sex steroid levels from the gonads. Negative feedback of the sex steroids onto the thymus inhibits release of thymosins including B_4 shutting off pituitary release of gonodotropins. Decrease in thymosins alters immune response and is especially effective in reducing suppressor T-cell function.

14.2 The Hypothalamic-Pituitary-Adrenal-Thymic (HPAT) Axis

Glucocorticoids regulate lymphocyte action, thymic structure and function and are themselves regulated by adrenocorticotropic hormone (ACTH) from the pituitary. We thus have a regulatory axis consisting of the hypothalamus, pituitary, adrenal and thymus. According to this scheme (Fig. 6) negative feedback of cortisol (corticosterone in rats) at the level of the hypothalamus-pituitary reduces the amount of ACTH released and subsequently decreases the amount of glucocorticoids secreted by the adrenal cortex.

The glucocorticoid also depresses thymic function resulting in a decrease in thymic weight and possibly a reduction in thymosin secretion. Decreasing thymosin should conceivably reduce T-lymphocyte function and furthermore glucocorticoids can exort a direct influence on T-lymphocytes via glucocorticoid receptors. Regulation of thymosin B_4 by the HPAT axis has not as yet been studied; however, thymectomy of mice at three days of age has been shown to reduce circulating levels of corticosterone [338] suggesting that a thymic factor can alter adrenal function. Whether this effect of thymus on adrenal is mediated through negative feedback at the hypothalamus-pituitary remains to be elucidated.

Of extreme interest is the recent report by Besedovsky et al. [260] showing that human peripheral blood lymphocytes in mixed lymphocyte culture produced a glucocorticoid increasing factor (GIF). GIF elevated corticosterone levels four fold and also increased ACTH but did not function in the absence of a pituitary. Thus, peripheral blood lymphocytes are able to produce a factor that probably stimulates a direct release of ACTH from the pituitary gland.

The HPAT axis also conceivably interact with the HPGT axis since cortico-releasing factor (CRF) injected into the lateral ventricules of gonadectomized/adrenalectomized rats inhibited LH but not FSH secretion [388]. Adrenalectomy has also been shown to suppress GnRH and LH secretions through some as yet unknown neurally mediated mechanism [389].

14.3 The Pineal-Hypothalamic-Pituitary (PHP) Axis

Pineal regulation of circadian rhythm is a confirmed fact (Fig. 6). Melatonin synthesized and released by the pineal in the dark suppresses GnRH as well as CRF from the hypothalamus and inhibits LH and ACTH release from the pituitary. This in turn depresses gonadal and adrenal function during the dark phase. Conversly thymosin α_1 is elevated in the dark possibly via interactions of the HPGT and HPAT axes.

14.4 Other Hormonal Axes That May Effect Immune Responses

Since thyroid hormones regulate immune function, possibly the hypothalamic-pituitary-thyroid axes may play a role in lymphocyte action. Growth hormone certainly effects lymphocytes and thymus, and GH is reduced as a result of thymectomy [338-340] suggesting some kind of thymosin-GH regulatory axis exists. Immune regulation of other important hormones such as prolactin must be examined.

15 Closing Remarks

T and B lymphocytes are effector cells of the cell mediated and humoral immune systems. B lymphocytes differentiated into plasma cells manufacture and secrete immunoglobin while subpopulations of T-lymphocytes are responsible either directly or indirectly for all aspects of the immune response. Immunological functions regulated or carried out by T-lymphocytes include delayed hypersensitivity reactions, graft tissue rejection, viral growth inhibition, and regulation of immunoglobulin production and tolerance [1-6]. Furthermore, interactions of the HPGT axis strongly effect reproductive behavior, levels of circulating sex and adrenal steroids and neuroendocrine interactions [383, 390-395]. Conceivably, interaction of the HPA and HPAT axis also play an important role in immune regulation because the glucocorticoids are potent immunoinhibitory/immunostimulatory substances.

One major factor that may strongly effect immune response and the function of the various immunoregulatory axes (HPGT, HPAT axes) is circadian rhythm. If immune responsiveness is altered as a result of circadian rhythm as has been suggested than humans exposed to altered light-dark regimes may potentially be at high risk of contracting diseases. The observation that immune reactivity is increased during the dark phase when cortisol is depressed and thymosin elevated may account for spiking fevers which occur in the evening. Furthermore, some medications might prove to be more effective if given to patients during the dark phase as a result of synergistic interactions with the increased immune response. Also alterations in light cycle in a hospital environment might conceivably increase immune responsiveness and facilitate patient recovery. If we could learn to effectively manipulate the systems responsible for regulation of the immune response we could better control graft rejection, autoimmune disease and the bodies ability to fight infection. With the major advances being made in the field to immunoregulation it is hoped that we may reach this goal in the next decade.

16 Acknowledgment

The authors gratefully wish to acknowledge the assistance of Ms. J. Oscher, Ms. B. Cromer and Ms. P. Short in the preparation of this manuscript.

17 References

1. Bowry, T. R.: Immunology simplified. Oxford Univ Press, Ibaden Delhi (1977)
2. Hood, L. E., Weissman, I. L., Wood, W. B.: Immunology. Benjamin/Cummings, Menlo Park, CA (1980)
3. Barett, J. T.: Basic Immunologhy and its medical application (2nd ed). C. V. Mosby, St. Louis, MO (1980)
4. Kimball, J. W.: Introduction to Immunology. MacMillan, New York (1983)
5. Barett, J. T.: Textbook of Immunology (3rd ed). C. V. Mosby, St. Louis, MO (1978)
6. Clark, W. R.: The experimental foundations of modern immunology (2nd ed). John Wiley & Sons, New York (1983)
7. Grossman, C. J., Sholiton, L. J., Roselle, G. A.: Estradiol regulation of thymic lymphocyte function in the rat. Mediation by serum thymic factors. J Ster Biochem, *16*, 683 (1982)
8. Grossman, C. J., Roselle, G. A.: The interrelationship of the HPG-thymic axis and immune system regulation. J Ster Biochem, *19*, 461 (1983)
9. Grossman, C. J., Sholiton, L. J., Roselle, G. A.: Dihydrotestosterone regulation of thymocyte function in the rat: Mediation by serum factors. J Ster Biochem, *19*, 1459 (1983)
10. Grossman, C. J.: The regulation of the immune system by sex steroids. Endo Rev, *5*, 435 (1984)
11. Grossman, C. J.: Gonadol steroids and immune response. Science, *227*, 257 (1985)
12. Low, T. L. K., Thurman, G. B., Zatz, M. M., Hu, S. K., Goldstein, A. L.: A multifaceted role for thymosin and its composite peptides in T-cell regulation. In: Advances in Immunopharmacol, Hadden J. (ed). Pergamon Press, New York, Page 67 (1981)
13. Ahlqvist, J.: Endocrine influences on the lymphatic organs, immune responses, inflammation and autoimmunity. Acta Endocrinol. (Suppl), *83*, 206 (1976)

14. Besedovsky, H., Sorkin, E.: Network of immunoneuroendocrine interactions. Clin Exp Immunol, *27*, 1 (1977)
15. Receptors and Hormone Action, Vol. I, O'Molley, B. W., Birnbaumer (ed), Academic Press, New York, San Francisco, London (1977)
16. Receptors and Hormone Action, Vol. II, O'Molley, B. W., Birnbaumer (ed), Academic Press, New York, San Francisco, London (1978)
17. Receptors and Hormone Action, Vol. III, Birnbaumer, L., O'Malley, B. W. (ed), Academic Press, New York, San Francisco, London (1978)
18. Receptors and Mechanism of Action of Steroid Hormones, Part II, Pasqualini, J. R. (ed) Marcel Dekker, Inc., New York, Basel (1977)
19. Grossman, C. J., Sholiton, L. J., Nathan, P.: Rat thymic estrogen receptor: I. Preparation, location and physiochemical properies. J Ster Biochem, *11*, 1233 (1979)
20. Grossman, C. J., Sholiton, L. J., Blaha, G. C., Nathan, P.: Rat thymic estrogen receptor. II Physiological properties. J Ster Biochem, *11*, 1241 (1979)
21. Reichman, M. E., Villee, C. A.: Estradiol binding by rat thymus cytosol. J Ster Biochem, *9*, 637 (1978)
22. Screpanti, I., Gulino, A., Pasquolini, J. R.: The fetal thymus of guinea pig as an estrogen target organ. Endocrinol, *111*, 1552 (1982)
23. Thompson, Jr., E. A.: The effects of estradiol upon the thymus of the exually immature female mouse. J Ster Biochem, *14*, 167 (1981)
24. Grossman, C. J., Nathan, P., Taylor, B. B., Sholiton, L. J.: Rat thymic dihydrotestosterone receptor: preparation, location and physiochemical properties. Steroids, *34*, 539 (1979)
25. Danel, L., Sovweine, G., Monier, J. C., Saez, S.: Specific estrogen binding sites in human lymphoid cells and thymus cells. J Ster Biochem, *18*, 559 (1983)
26. Grossman, C. J., Soliton, L. J., Helmsworth, J. A.: Characteristics of the cytoplasmic and nuclear dihydrotestosterone receptors of rat and human thymic tissue. Steroids, *42*, 11 (1983)
27. Gulino, A., Screpanti, I., Torrisi, M. R., Frati, L.: Estrogen receptors and estrogen sensitivity of fetal thymocytes are restricted to blast lymphoid cells. Endocrinol, *117*, 47 (1985)
28. Sasson, S., Mayer, M.: Effect of androgenic steroids on rat thymus and thymocytes in suspension. J Ster Biochem, *14*, 509 (1981)
29. McCruden, A. B., Stimson, W. H.: Androgen binding cytosol receptors in the rat thymus: physiochemical properties, specificity and localization. Thymus, *3*, 105 (1981)
30. Pearce, P. T., Khalid, B. A. K., Funder, J. W.: Progesterone receptors in rat thymus. Endocrinol, *113*, 1287 (1983)
31. Pearce, P., Khalid, B. A. K., Funder, J. W.: Androgens and the thymus. Endocrinol *109*, 1073 (1981)
32. Sullivan, D. A., Wira, C. R.: Sex hormone and glucocorticoid receptors in the bursa of Fabricius of immature chicks. J Immunol, *122*, 2617 (1979)
33. Wira, C. R., Munck, A.: Glucocorticoid-receptor complexes in rat thymus cells. J Biolog Chem, *249*, 5328 (1974)
34. Munck. A., Brinck-Johnson, T.: Specific and nonspecific physiochemical interactions of glucocorticoid and related steroids with rat thymus cells *in vitro*. J Biolog Chem, *243*, 5556 (1968)
35. Wira, C., Munck, A.: Specific glucocorticoid receptors in thymus cells. J Biolog Chem, *245*, 3436 (1970)
36. Schaumburg, B. P.: Studies of the glucocorticoid-binding protein from thymocytes. Biochem Biophy Acta, *214*, 520 (1970)
37. Bell, P. A., Munck, A.: Steroid-binding properties and stabilization of cytoplasmic glucocorticoid receptors from rat thymus cells. Biochem J, *136*, 97 (1973)
38. Schaumburg, B. P., Bojesen, E.: Specifity and thermodynamic properties of the corticosteroid binding to a receptor of rat thymocytes *in vitro*. Biochem Biophy Acta *170*, 172 (1968)
39. Sloman, J. C., Bell, P. A.: The dependence of specific nuclear binding of glucocorticoids by rat thymus cells on cellular ATP levels. Biochem Biophy Acta, *428*, 403 (1976)
40. Eidinger, D., Garrett, T. J.: Studies of the regulatory effects of the sex hormones on antibody formation and stem cell differentiation. J Exp Med, *136*, 1098 (1972)
41. Phuc, L. H., Papiernik, M., Dardenne, M.: Thymic involution in pregnant mice. II Functional aspects of the remaining thymocytes. Clin Exp Immunol, *44*, 253 (1981)

42. Phuc, L. M., Papiernick, M., Berrich, S., Duval, D.: Thymic involution in pregnant mice. I Characterization of the remaining thymocyte population. Clin Exp Immunol, *44*, 247 (1981)
43. Millar, K. G., Mills, P., Baines, M. G.: A study of the influence of pregnancy on the thymus gland of the mouse. Am J Obstet Gynecol, *117*, 913 (1973)
44. Low, T. L. K., Thurman, G. B., McAdoo, M., McClure, J., Rossio, L., Naylor, P. H., Goldstein, A. L.: The chemistry and biology of thymosin. J Biol Chem, *254*, 981 (1979)
45. Low, T. L. K., Hu, S-K., Goldstein, A. L.: Complete amino acid sequence of bovine thymosin B_4. Proc Nat Acad Sci, *78*, 1162 (1981)
46. Robinson, G. A., Butcher, R. W., Sutherland, E. W.: Cyclic AMP. Academic Press, New York (1971)
47. Birnbaumer, L.: The action of hormones and nucleotides on membrane bound adenylcyclase: an overview. In: Receptors and Hormone Action, Vol I, O'Malley, B. W., Birnbaumer, 0. (ed), Academic Press, New York, San Francisco, London, Pages 485–547, (1974)
48. Naylor, P. H., Sheppard, H., Thurman, G. B., Goldstein, A. L.: Increase of cyclic GMP induced in murine thymocytes by thymosin fraction 5. Biomed. Biophy Res Comm, *73*, 843 (1976)
49. Garaci, C. R., Torrisi, M. R., Jezzi, T., Frati, L., Goldstein, A. L., Garaci, E.: Receptors for thymosin alpha 1 on mouse thymocytes. Cell Immunol, *91*, 289 (1985)
50. Lesniak, M. A., Roth, J. A.: Regulation of receptor concentration by homologous hormone. Effects of human growth hormone on its receptor in IM-9 lymphocytes. J Biolog Chem, *251*, 3729 (1976)
51. Arrenbrecht, S.: Specific binding of growth hormone to thymocytes. Nature, *252*, 255 (1974)
52. Bhathena, S. J., Gazdar, H. F., Schechter, G. P., Russell, E. K., Soehnlen, F. E., Gritsman, A., Recant, L.: Expression of glucagon receptors on T- and B-lymphoblasts: comparison with insulin receptors. Endocrinol, *111*, 684 (1982)
53. Krug, V., Krug, F., Cuatrecasos, P.: Emergence of insulin receptors on human lymphocytes during in vitro transformation. Proc Natl Acad Sci USA, *69*, 2604 (1972)
54. Helderman, J. H., Strom, T. B.: Specific insulin binding site on T and B lymphocytes as a marker of cell activation. Nature, *274*, 62 (1978)
55. Strom, T. B., Helderman, J. H., Williams, R. M.: Rapid murine mixed lymphocyte cultures assessed by emergence of T-cell insulin receptors. Proc Clin Diab Transplant For, *7*, 148 (1977)
56. Helderman, J. H., Strom, T. B.: Emergence of insulin receptors upon alloimmune T-cells in the rat. J Clin Invest, *59*, 338 (1977)
57. Gulino, A., Screpanti, I., Pasqualini, J. R.: Estrogen and antiestrogen effects on different lymphoid cell populations in the developing fetal thymus of guinea pig. Endocrinol, *113*, 1754 (1983)
58. Batchelor, J. R.: Hormonal control of antibody formation. In: Regulation of the antibody response. Cinader, B. (ed), Charles C. Thomas, Springfield, IL Page 276 (1968)
59. Tartakovsky, B., DeBaetselies, P., Feldman, M., Segal, S.: Sex associated differences in the immune response against fetal major histocompatibility antigens. Transplant, *32*, 395 (1981)
60. Butterworth, M. B., McClellan, B., Alansmith, M.: Influence of sex on immunoglobin levels. Nature (Lond), *214*, 1224 (1967)
61. Rhodes, K., Scott, A., Markham, R. L., Monk-Jones, M. E.: Immunological sex differences. A study of patients with rheumatoid arthritis, their relatives and controls. Ann Rheum Dis, *28*, 104 (1969)
62. Rowley, M. J., Mackay, I. R.: Measurement of antibody producing capacity in man. Clin Exp Immunol, *5*, 407 (1969)
63. Ainbender, E., Weisinger, R., Hevizy, M., Hodes, H. L.: Difference in immunoglobulin class of polio antibody in the serum of men and women. J Immunol, *101*, 1 (1968)
64. Wira, C. R., Sandoe, C. P.: Hormonal regulation of immunoglobulins: infuence of estradiol on immunoglobulins A and G in the rat uterus. Endocrinol, *106*, 1020 (1980)
65. Sullivan, D. A., Wira, C. R.: Hormonal regulation of immunoglobulins in the rat uterus: uterine response to multiple estradiol treatments. Endocrinol, *114*, 650 (1984)
66. Jerne, N. K., Norden, A. A., Henry, C.: The agar plaque technique for recognizing antibody producing cells. Cell-Bound Antibodies, Wistar, Philadelphia, Page 109 (1963)
67. Blazkovec, A. A., Orsini, M. W., Maginn, P. C.: Sexual dimorphism in the primary immune response of the syrian hamster. Int Arch Allergy App Immunol, *44*, 274 (1973)

68. Orsini, M. W., Blazkovec, A. A.: Sexual dimorphism in the secondary immune response of the syrian hamsters. Int Arch Allergy App Immunol, *46*, 858 (1974)
69. Terres, G., Morrison, S. L., Habicht, G. S.: A quantitative difference in the immune response between male and female mice. Pro Soc Exp Biol Med, *27*, 664 (1968)
70. Batchelor, J. R., Chapman, B. A.: The influence of sex upon the antibody response to an incompatible tumor. Immunol, *9*, 553 (1965)
71. Graff, R. J., Hildemann, W. H., Snell, G. D.: Histocompatibility genes of mice. Transplant, *4*, 425 (1966)
72. Graff, R. J., Lappe, M. A., Snell, G. D.: The influence of the gonads and adrenal glands on the immune response to skin grafts. Transplant, *7*, 105 (1969)
73. Gross, L.: Influence of sex on the evolution of a transplantable mouse sarcoma. Pro Soc Exp Biol Med, *47*, 273 (1941)
74. Gross, L.: Influence of sex on resistance to interperistoneal inoculation of sarcoma in mice. Proc Soc Exp Biol Med, *49*, 67 (1942)
75. Raveche, E., Klassen, L. W., Steinberg, A. D.: Sex differences in formation of anti-T-cell antibodies. Nature, *263*, 415 (1976)
76. Roubinian, J. R., Papoian, R., Talal, N.: Androgenic hormones modulate auto-antibody responses and improve survival in murine lupus. J Clin Invest, *59*, 1066 (1977)
77. Roubinian, J. R., Talal, N., Greenspan, J. S., Goodman, J. R., Siiteri, P. K.: Effects of castration and sex hormone treatment on survival, anti-nucleic acid antibodies, and glomerulonephritis in NZB/NZW F_1 mice. J Exp Med, *147*, 1568 (1978)
78. Roubinian, J. R., Talal, N., Greenspan, J. S., Goodman, J. R., Siiteri, P. K.: Delayed androgen treatment prolongs survival in murine lupus. J Clin Invest, *63*, 902 (1979)
79. Roubinian, J. R., Talal, N., Siiteri, P. K., Sadakin, J. A.: Sex hormone modulation of autoimmunity in NZB/NZW mice. Arth Rheum, *22*, 1162 (1979)
80. Calzolori, A.: Rescherches experimentales sus un rapport probable entre la function du thymus et celle des testicules. Arch Itol Biol, *30*, 71 (1898)
81. Chiodi, H.: The relationship between the thymus and the sexual organs. Endocrinol, *26*, 107 (1940)
82. Castro, J. E.: Orchidectomy and the immune response. I. Effect of orchidectomy on lymphoid tissue of mice. Proc R Soc (Lond), *185*, 425 (1974)
83. Chiodi, H.: Thymus hypertrophy induced by castration in old male rats and ice. Fed Proc, *35*, 277 (abstract 395) (1976)
84. Castro, J. E.: Immunological and anti-tumor effects of orchidectomy. In: Immunological influences on human fertility, Boettcher, B. (ed). Proceedings of the workshop on Fertility in Human Reproduction. Aca NY, Page 295 (1977)
85. Streng, C. B., Nathan, P.: The immune response in steroid deficient mice. Immunol, *24*, 559 (1973)
86. Evans, H. M., Simpson, M. E.: Reduction of the thymus by gonadotropic hormone. Anat Rec, *60*, 423 (1934)
87. Castro, J. E.: Orchidectomy and the immune response. II. Response of orchideceomized mice to antigen. Proc R Soc (Lond), *185*, 437 (1974)
88. Castro, J. E.: Immunological effects of orchidectomy. Br J Urol, *47*, 89 (1975)
89. Yohn, D. S.: Sex related resistance in hamsters to adenovirus oncogenesis. Prog Exp Tumor Res, *18*, 138 (1973)
90. Fong, C. K. Y., Ledinko, N.: Enhancement by estrogen of adenovirus or spontaneous transformation of hamster cells in culture. Cancer Res, *30*, 889 (1970)
91. Franks, C. R., Perkins, F. T., Bishop, D.: The effect of sex hormones on the growth of Hela tumor nodules in male and female mice. Br J Cancer, *31*, 100 (1975)
92. Stern, K., Davidsohn, I.: Effect of estrogen and cortisone on immune hemoantibody in mice of inbred strain. J Immunol, *74*, 479 (1955)
93. Von Haam, E., Rosenfeld, I.: The effect of estrone on antibody production. J Immunol, *43*, 109 (1942)
94. Kenny, J. F., Gray, J. A.: Sex differences in immunological response. Studies of antibody production by individual speen cells after stimulus with Escherichia coli antigen. Pediatr Res, *5*, 246 (1971)

95. Visilakis, G. J., Kunz, H. W., Gill, T. J.: The effect of gonadectomy on antibody production by inbred rats. Int Arch Allergy Appl Immunol, *47*, 730 (1974)
96. Gill, T. J., Kuntz, H. W.: Genetic and cellular factors in the immune response. II. Evidence for polygenic control of the antibody response from further breeding studies and from pedigree analysis. J Immunol, *106*, 980 (1971)
97. Maor, D., Englander, T., Eylan, E., Alexander, P.: Participation of hormone in the early stages of the immune response. Acta Endocrinol, *75*, 205 (1974)
98. Paavonen, T., Anderson, L. C., Adlercreutz, H.: Sex hormone regulation of *in vitro* immune response. Estradiol enhances human B-cell maturation via inhibition of suppressor T-cells in pokeweed mitogen-stimulated cultures. J Exp Med, *154*, 1935 (1981)
99. Kappas, A., Jones, H. E. H., Roitt, I. M.: Affects of sex hormones on immunological phenomena. Nature, *198*, 902 (1963)
100. Lurie, M. B., Harris, T. N., Abramson, S., Allison, J. M.: Constitutional factors in resistance to infection. II. The effect of estrogen on tubercuin skin sensitivity and on the allergy of the internal tissues. Am Rev Tuberculo, *59*, 186 (1949)
101. Kalland, T., Forsberg, J. G.: Delayed hypersensitivity response to oxazolone in neonatally estrogenized mice. Cancer Lett, *4*, 141 (1978)
102. Waltman, S. R., Burde, R. M., Berrios, J.: Prevention of corneal homograft rejection by estrogens. Transplant, *11*, 194 (1971)
103. Kalland, T., Strand, O., Forsberg, J. G.: Long-term effects of neonatal estrogen treatment on mitogen responsiveness of mouse spleen lymphocytes. J Clin Invest, *63*, 413 (1979)
104. Stimson, W. H., Hunter, I. C.: An investigation into the immunosuppressive properties of estrogen. J Endocrinol, *69*, 42P (1976)
105. Seaman, W. E., Gindhart, T. D.: Effect of estrogen on natural killer cells. Arth Rheum, *22*, 1234 (1979)
106. Morishima, A., Henrich, R.: Lymphocyte transformation and oral contraceptives. Lancet (Sept), *14*, 646 (1974)
107. Ablin, R. J., Bruns, G. R., Guinan, P. D., Sheik, H. A., Bush, I. M.: Hormal therapy and alteration of lymphocyte proliferation. J Lab Clin Med, *87*, 227 (1976)
108. Ablin, R. J., Bhatti, R. A., Guianan, P. D., Khin, W.: Modulatory effects of oestrogen on immunological responsiveness. II. Suppression of tumor-associated immunity in patients with prostatic cancer. Clin Exp Immunol *38*, 83 (1979)
109. Ablin, R. J., Bruns, G. R. Guinan, P. D., Bush, I. M.: Diethylstilbestrol exposure and lymphocyte impairment. J Am Med Asso, *292*, 1863 (1974)
110. Mandybur, T. I., Ormsby, I., Buncher, C. R.: Enhanced development of mammory tumors in rats following transplacenta and neonata exposure to ethylnitrosourea. Cancer Res, *38*, 3182 (1978)
111. Moon, R. C., Fricks, C. M.: Influence of gonadal hormones and age on 1,2 dimethylhydrozine — induced colon carcinogenesis. Cancer, *40*, 2502 (1977)
112. Taper, H. S.: The effect of estradiol 17-phenylpropionate and estradiol benzoate on N-nitrosomorpholine induced liver carcinogenesis in ovariectomized female rats. Cancer, *42*, 462 (1978)
113. Brown, C. E., Warren, S., Chute, R. N., Ryan, K. J., Todd, R. B.: Hormonally induced tumors of the reproductive system of parabiosed male rats. Cancer Res, *39*, 3971 (1979)
114. Warren, S., Brown, C. E., Chute, R. N.: Is breast cancer a result of endocrine targeting? (How women differ from rats or mice). Ann Clin Lab Sci, *9*, 87 (1979)
115. Sekiya, S., Kikuchi, Y., Katoh, I., Kobayoshi, W., Takeda, B., Tokamizawa, J.: Effect of ovariectomy, adrenelectomy and hypophysectomy on carcinogenesis of the endometrium by 7,12-dimethylbenz [a] anthrace in rats. Gynecol Oncol, *7*, 281 (1979)
116. Kittas, C., Henry, L.: Effect of sex hormones on the immune system of guinea-pigs and on the development of toxoplasmic lesions in non-lymphoid organs. Clin Exp Immunol, *36*, 16 (1979)
117. Kittas, C., Henry, L.: Effect of sex hormones on the response of mice to infection with Toxoplasma gondii. Br J Exp Path, *61*, 590 (1980)
118. Talal, N.: Systemic lupus erythematosis, autoimmunity, sex and inheritance. Letter to the Editor, New Eng J Med, *301*, 838 (1979)
119. Horowitz, S., Borcherding, W., Vishnu, M. A., Chesney, R., Schulte-Wisserman, H., Hong, R.: Induction of suppressor T-cells in systemic lupus erythematosis by thymosin and cultured thymic epithelium. Science, *197*, 999 (1977)

120. Lahita, R. G., Bradlow, H. L., Kunkel, H. G., Fishman, J.: Increased 16 alpha-hydroxylation of estradiol in systemic lupus erythematosus. J Clin Endo Met, *53*, 174 (1981)
121. Lahita, R. G., Bradlow, H. L., Kunkel, H. G., Fishman, J.: Alterations of estrogen metabolism in systemic lupus erythematosus. Arth Rheum, *22*, 1195 (1979)
122. Miller, K. B., Schwartz, R. S.: Familial abnormalities of suppressor-cell function in systemic lupus erythematosus. N Eng J Med, *301*, 803 (1979)
123. Raveche, E. S., Tjio, J. H., Steinberg, A. D.: Studies of the effects of sex hormones on autosomal and x-linked genetic control of induced and spontaneous antibody production. Arth Rheum, 22, 1177 (1979)
124. Cohn, D. A.: High sensitivity to androgen as a contributing factor in sex differences in the immune response. Arth Rheum *22*, 1218 (1979)
125. Steinberg, A. D., Melez, K. A., Raveche, E. S., Reeves, J. P., Boegel, W. A., Smathers, P. A., Taurog, J. D., Weinlein, L., DuVic, M.: Approach to the study of the role of sex hormones in autoimmunity. Arth Rheum, *22*, 1170 (1979)
126. Weiner, L.: Possible role of androgen receptors in amyotrophic lateral sclerosis. Arch Neurol, *37*, 129 (1980)
127. Arnason, B. G., Richman, D. P.: Effect of oral contraceptives on experimental demyelinating disease. Arch Neurol, *21*, 103 (1969)
128. Brown, J. B.: Urinary excretion of estrogens during pregnancy, lactation, and reestablishment of menstruation. Lancet, *1*, 707 (1956)
129. Miller, H. G., Schepira, K.: Etiological aspects of multiple sclerosis. Brit Med J, *17*, 37 (1959)
130. Miller, J.: The influence of pregnancy or disseminated sclerosis. Proc Royal Soc Med, *54*, 4 (1961)
131. Frank, M.: Effect of sex hormones on the complement related clinical disorder of hereditary angioedema. Arth Rheum, *22*, 1295 (1979)
132. Gadek, J., Hosea, S., Grelfand, J., Frank, M.: Response of variant hereditary angioedema phenotypes to danazol therapy: genetic implications. J Clin Invest, *64*, 280 (1979)
133. Harris, R.: Coccidioidomycosis complicating pregnancy. Obst Gynec, *28*, 401 (1966)
134. Drutz, D., Huppert, M., Sun, S., McGuire, W.: Human sex hormones stimulate the growth and maturation of coccidioides immitus. Inf Immunity, *32*, 897 (1981)
135. Drutz, D., Catanzaro, A.: Coccidioidomycosis. Am Review of Resp Dis, *117*, 727 (1978)
136. Walzer, P., Powell, R.: Experimental pneumocystis carinii infection in nude and steroid treated normal mice: Proceedings of the Third International Workshop in Nude: 123 (1982)
137. Freeman, D., Barno, A.: Deaths from Asian influenza associated with pregnancy. Am J Obstet Gynecol, *78*, 1172 (1959)
138. Smale, L., Waechter, K.: Dissemination of coccidioidomycosis in pregnancy. Am J Obstet Gynecol, *107*, 356 (1970)
139. Stobo, J., Paul, S., VanScoy, R., Hermans, P.: Suppressor thymus derived lymphocytes in fungal infection. J Clin Invest, *57*, 319 (1976)
140. London, W.: Sex differences in response to Hepatitis-B virus. Arth Rheum, *22*, 1258 (1979)
141. Blumberg, B.: Sex differences in response to Hepatitis-B virus. Arth Rheum, *22*, 1261 (1979)
142. Lederman, M.: Cell-mediated immunity and pregnancy. Chest, *86*, 6S (1984)
143. Spector, S.: Reciprocal relationship between preganacy and pulmonary disease. Chest, *86*, 1S (1984)
144. Catanzaro, A.: Pulmonary mycoses in pregnant women Chest, *86*, 14S (1984)
145. Luft, B., Remington, J.: Effect of pregnancy on augmentation of natural kiler cell activity by carinii bacterium parvum and toxiplasma gondii. J Immunol, *132*, 2375 (1984)
146. Snider, D.: Pregnancy and tuberculosis Chest, *86*, 10S (1984)
147. Tanaka, A., Hirota, K., Takahashi, K., Numazaki, Y.: Suppression of cell-mediated immunity to cytomegalo virus and tubercuin in pregnancy employing the leukocyte migration inhibition test. Micro Immunol, *27*, 937 (1983)
148. Duncan, M., Pearson, J.: The association of pregnancy and leprosy. III. Erythema nodosum leprosum in pregnancy and lactation. Leprosy Reviews, *55*, 129 (1984)
149. Greenberg, M., Jacobziner, H., Pakter, J., Weisl, B.: Maternal mortality in the epidemic of Asian influenza, New York City, 1957. Am J Obstet Gynec, *76*, 897 (1958)
150. Public Health Laboratory Statistics, Brit M J, *2*, 915 (1958)

151. Friedman, D., Netti, F., Schreiber, A.: Effect of estradiol and steroid analogs on the clearance of immunoglobulin G-coated erythrocytes. J Clin Invest *75*, 162–167 (1985)
152. Buyon, J., Korchak, H., Rutherford, L., Ganguly, M., Weissman, G.: Female hormones reduce neutrophil responsiveness *in vitro*. Arth Rheum *27*, 623–630 (1984)
153. Cohn, D. A.: Sensitivity to androgen. A possible factor in sex differences in the immune response. Clin Exp Immunol *38*, 218 (1979)
154. Franks, C. R.: Hormonal exposure and lymphocyte impairment. J Am Med Assoc *232*, 19 (1975)
155. Skowron-Cendrzak, A., Plonka, I., Bubak, M., Rembiesa, R.: Reduction of the graft-versus-host reactivity of mouse and rat spleen cells by 5-androstone-3,17-dione. Folia Biol (Praha) *12*, 190 (1975)
156. Blazovec, A. A., Orsini, M. W.: Ontogenic aspects of sexual dimorphism and the primary immune response to sheep erythrocytes in hamsters from prepuberty to senescence. Int Arch Allergy App Immunol *50*, 55 (1976)
157. Hirota, Y., Suzuki, T., Chazono, Y., Bito, Y.: Humoral immune response characteristics of testosterone propionat e treated chicks. Immunol *30*, 341 (1970)
158. Szenberg, A.: Influence of testosterone on the primary lymphoid organs of the chicken. In: Wolstenholme, G. E., Knight, J. (eds.). Hormones and the Immune System, Ciba Foundation Study Group No. 35, Ed: Churchill, London, p 42 (1970)
159. Dixon, D. K., Fitzsimmons, R. C.: Thymic development of the chick embryo as influenced by hormonal and early surgical bursectomy. Dev Comp Immunol *4*, 713 (1980)
160. Hirota, Y., Suzuki, T., Bito, Y.: The B-cell development independent of bursa of Fabricius but dependent upon the thymus in chickens treated with testosterone propionate. Immunol *39*, 37 (1980)
161. Hirota, Y., Suzuki, T., Bito, Y.: The development of unusual B-cell functions in the testosterone-propionate-treated chicken. Immunol *39*, 29 (1980)
162. Kotani, M., Nowa, Y., Fujii, H., Fukumoto, T., Tsuchiya, H.: Histological observations of inhibitory effects of testosterone on lymphoid regeneration in the thymus-independent areas of B-mice. Arch Histol Jap *38*, 117 (1975)
163. Kotani, M., Nawa, Y., Fujii, H.: Inhibition by testosterone of immune reactivity and of lymphoid regeneration in irradiated and marrow reconstituted mice. Experientica *30*, 1343 (1974)
164. Fujii, H., Nowa, Y., Tsuchiya, H., Matsuno, K., Fukumoto, T., Fukuda, S., Kotani, M.: Effect of a single administration of testosterone on the immune response and lymphoid tissue in mice. Cell Immunol *20*, 315 (1975)
165. Verheul, H. A. M., Stimson, W. H., Den Hollander, F. C., Schuurs, H. H. W. M.: The effect of nandrolene, testosterone, and their decanoate esters on murine lupus. Clin Exp Immunol *44*, 11 (1981)
166. Raveche, E. S., Tjio, J. H., Steinberg, A. D.: Genetic studies in NZB mice. IV. The effect of sex hormones on the spontaneous production of anti-T cell antibodies. Arth Rheum *23*, 48 (1980)
167. Laskin, C. A., Taurog, J. D., Smathers, P. A., Steinberg, A. D.: Studies of defective tolerance in murine lupus. J Immunol *127*, 1743 (1981)
168. Talal, N.: Sex steroid hormones and systemic lupus erythymatosus. Arth Rheum *24*, 1054 (1981)
169. Inman, R. D.: Immunological sex differences and the female predominance in systemic lupus erythematosus. Arth Rheum *21*, 657 (1978)
170. Sakans, T., Steinberg, A. D., Green, I.: Studies of immune functions of patients with systemic lupus erythematosus. I. Dysfunction of suppressor T-cell activity related to impaired generation of, rather than response to, suppressor cells. Arth Rheum *21*, 657 (1978)
171. Morimoto, C.: Loss of suppressor T-lymphocyte function in patients with systemic lupus erythematosus (SLE). Clin Exp Immunol *32*, 125 (1978)
172. Wingrave, S. J.: Reduction in incidence of rheumatoid arthritis associated with oral contraceptives. Lancet *1*, 569 (1978)
173. Linos, A., Worthington, J. W., O'Fallon, W. M., Kurland, L. T.: The epidemiology of rheumatoid arthritis in Rochester, Minnesota: A study of prevalence, incidence, and mortality. Am J Epidemiol *111*, 87 (1980)
174. Vandenbroucke, J. P., Valkenburg, H. A., Boersma, J. W.: Oral contraceptives and rheumatoid arthritis: further evidence for a preventive effect. Lancet ii, 839 (1982)
175. Vondenbroucke, J. P.: Rheumatoid arthritis, the pill and self selection. Lancet ii, 1282 (1982)

176. Okayasu, I., Kong, Y. M., Rose, N. R.: Effect of castration and sex hormones on experimental autoimmune thyroiditis. Clin Immunol Immun Path *20*, 240 (1981)
177. Gerretsen, G., Kremer, J., Nater, J. P., Bleumink, E., de Gast, C. C., The, T. T.: Immune reactivity of women on hormonal contraceptives. Dinitrochlorobenzene sensitization test and skin reactivity to irritants. Contracept *19*, 83 (1979)
178. Gerretsen, G., Kremer, J., Bleumink, E., Nater, J. P., de Gast, C. C., The, T. T.: Immune reactivity of women on hormonal contraceptives. Phytochemagglutinin and concanavalin-A induced lymphocyte response. Contracept *22*, 25 (1980)
179. Gelfond, J. A.: Exploring sex for therapeutic purposes. N Eng J Med *23*, 1417 (1983)
180. Ann, Y. S., Harrington, W. J., Simon, S. R., Mylvaganam, R., Pall, L. M., So, A. G.: Danazol for the treatment of idiopathic thrombocytopenic purpura. N Eng J Med *308*, 1396 (1983)
181. Loudon, W.: Sex differences in response to Hepatitis B virus. Arth Rheum *22*, 1267 (1979)
182. Shoupe, D., Lobo, R.: Insulin resistance in polycystic ovary syndrome. Fert Steril *147*, 588 (1983)
183. Shoupe, D., Lobo, R.: The influence of androgens on insulin resistance. Fert Steril *41*, 385 (1984)
184. Elder, M., Maclaren, N.: Identification of profound peripheral T-lymphocyte immunodeficiencies in the spontaneously diabetic BB rat. J Immunol *130*, 1723 (1983)
185. Guttmann, R., Colle, E., Michel, F., Seemayer, T.: Spontaneous diabetes mellitus syndrome in the rat. II. T-lymphopenia and its association with clinical disease and pancreatic lymphocytic infiltration. J Immunol *130*; 1732 (1983)
186. Gardner, F., Besa, E.: Physiologic mechanisms and the hematopoetic effects of the androstanes and their derivatives. Current Topics Hematol *4*, 123 (1983)
187. Ekman, P., Snochowski, M., Zetterberg, A., Hogberg, B., Gustafsson, J.: Steroid receptor content in human prostatic carcinoma and response to endocrine therapy. Cancer *44*, 1173 (1979)
188. Mendenhall, C., and the V. A. Cooperative Study Group: I. N Eng J Med *311*, 1464 (1984)
189. Kincl, F. A., Ciaccio, L. A.: Suppression of immune response by progesterone. Endocrinol Exp *14*, 27 (1980)
190. Sekiya, S., Kamiyama, M., Takamizawa, H.: *In vivo* and *in vitro* tests of inhibitory effect of progesterone on cellmediated immunity in rats bearing a syngenic uterine adenocarcinoma. J Nat Cancer Inst *54*, 769 (1975)
191. Mori, T., Kobayashi, H., Nishimura, T., Mori, T. S., Fujii, G., Inou, T.: Inhibitory effecty of progesterone on the phytohaemagglutinin-induced transformation of human peripheral lymphocytes. Immunol Commun *4*, 519 (1975)
192. Mori, T., Kobayashi, H., Nishimoto, H., Suzuki, A., Nishimura, T., Mori, T.: Inhibitory effect of progesterone and 20-hydroxy-pregn-4-en-3-one on the phytohaemagglutinininduced transformation of human lymphocytes. Am J Obstet Gynecol *127*, 151 (1977)
193. Holdstock, G., Chastenay, B. F., Krawitt, E. L.: Effcts of testosterone, estradiol and progesterone on immune regulation. Clin Exp Immunol *47*, 449 (1982)
194. Viklicky, V., Palackova, M., Vojtiskova, M., Draber, P., Kohda, M. E.: Immuno-suppressive effect of an antiandrogenic steroid (cyproterone acetate) in mice. Folio Biol (Praha) *23*, 145 (1977)
195. Neuman, F., Schleusener, A., Albring, M.: Pharmacology of antiandrogens. IV. Therapy and sex hormones and hormone metabolism. In: Hammerstein, J., Lochni, V., Neumann, Y., Plewig, G. (ed.). Androgenization in women, acne, seborrhoea, androgenetic alopaecia and hirsutism. Lectures and discussion of a symposium. Berlin, 23rd–24th Feeb. 1979. Excerpta Medica, Amsterdam, p 147 (1980)
196. Bardawil, W. A., Mitchell, G. W., McKeogh, R. P., Marchant, D. J.: Behavior of skin homografts in human pregnancy. I. Habitual abortion. Am J. Obstet Gynecol *84*, 1283 (1962)
197. Thong, Y. H., Steele, R. W., Vincent, M. M., Hensen, S. A., Bellanti, J. A.: Impaired *in vitro* cell-mediated immunity to rubella virus during pregnancy. N Eng J Med *289*, 604 (1971)
198. Finn, R., St. Hill, C. A., Govan, A. J., Ralfs, I. G., Gurney, F. J.: Immunological responsiveness in pregnancy and survival of fetal homograft. Br Med J *3*, 150 (1972)
199. Purtilo, D. T., Hallgren, H. M., Yunis, E. J.: Depressed maternal lymphocyte response to phytohemagglutinin in human pregnancy. Lancet *1*, 769 (April 8) (1972)
200. Smith, J. K., Caspary, E. A., Field, E. J.: Immune response in pregnancy. Lancet *1*, 96 (January 8) (1972)
201. Wyle, F. A., Kent, J. R.: Immunosuppression by sex steroid hormones. I. The effect upon PHA and PPD-stimulated lymphocytes. Clin Exp Immunol *27*, 407 (1977)

202. Anderson, R. H., Monroe, C. W.: Experimental study of the behavior of adult human skin homografts during pregnancy. Am J Obstet Gyn *84*, 1096 (1962)
203. Black, W. G., Simon, J., McNutt, S. H., Casida, L. E.: Investigations on the physiological basis for the differential response of estrous and pseudopregnant rabbit uteri to induced infection. Am J Vet Res *11*, 318 (1953)
204. Carter, J.: The effect of progesterone, oestradiol and HCG on cell-mediated immunity in pregnant mice. J Reprod Fertil *46*, 211 (1976)
205. Siiteri, P. K., Febres, F., Clemens, L. E., Chang, J. R., Gondos, B., Stites, D.: Progesterone and maintenance of pregnancy: is progesterone nature's immuno-suppressant? Ann NY Acad Sci *286*, 384 (1977)
206. Watnick, A. S., Russo, R. A.: Survival of skin homografts in uteri of pregnant progesterone-estrogen treated rats. Proc Soc Exp Biol Med *128*, 1 (1968)
207. Anderson, J. M.: Transplantation — nature's success. Lancet *2*, 1077 (November 3) (1971)
208. Anderson, J. M.: Studies of artificial immunological inertia. In: Anderson, J. M. (ed.). The Biology and Surgery of Tissue Transplantation, Oxford Press, London, p 129 (1970)
209. Simmons, R. L., Price, A. L., Ozerkis, A. J.: The immunologic problem of pregnancy. V. The effect of estrogen and progesterone on allograft survival. Am J Obstet Gyn *100*, 908 (1968)
210. Munroe, J. P.: Progesteroids as immunosuppressive agents. J Reticuloendothel Soc *9*, 361 (1971)
211. Mariyama, I., Sugawa, T.: Progesterone facilitates implantation of xenogenic cultured cells in hamster uteries. Nature New Biol *236*, 150 (1972)
212. Skinnides, L. F., Laxdal, V.: The effect of progesterone, oestrogens and hydrocortisone on the mitogenic response of lymphocytes to phytohaemagglutinin in pregnant and nonpregnant women. Br J Obst Gyn 88, 1110 (1981)
213. Mori, T., Kobayashi, H.: Possible role of progesterone in immunoregulation during pregnancy. In: Boettcher, B. (ed.). Immunological Influence on Human Fertility; Proceedings of the Workshop on Fertility in Human Reproduction. Academic Press, NY, p 175 (1977)
214. Stites, D. P., Pava, C. S., Clemens, L. E., Kuhn, R. W., Siiteri, P. K.: Immunologic regulation in pregnancy. Arth Rheum *22*, 1300 (1979)
215. Neifeld, J. P., Tormey, D. C.: Effect of steroid hormones on phytohemagglutinin-stimulated human peripheral blood lymphocytes. Trans *27*, 309 (1979)
216. Schiff, R. I., Mercier, D., Buckley, R. H.: Inability of gestational hormones to account for the inhibitory effects of pregnancy plasmas on lymphocyte responses *in vitro*. Cell Immunol *20*, 69 (1975)
217. Clemens, L. E., Siiteri, P. K., Stites, D. P.: Mechanism of immunosuppression of progesterone on maternal lymphocyte activation during pregnancy. J Immunol *122*, 1978 (1979)
218. Mendelsohn, J., Multer, M. M., Berheim, J. L.: Inhibition of human lymphocyte stimulation by steroid hormones. Cytokinetic Mechanisms. Clin Exp Immunol *27*, 127 (1977)
219. Stites, D., Bugbee, S., Siiteri, P.: Differential actions of progesterone and cortisol on lymphocyte and monocyte interaction during lymphocyte activation — relevance to immunosuppression in pregnancyi. J Repro Immunol *2*, 215 (1983)
220. Stites, D., Siiteri, P.: Steroids as immunosuppressants in pregnancy. Immunological Reviews *75*, 117 (1983)
221. Bigger, J. F., Palmberg, P. F., Becker, B.: Increased cellular sensitivity to glucocorticoids in primary openangle glaucoma. Invest Ophthal *11*, 832 (1972)
222. Yu, T. Y. D., Kacena, A., Pearson, C. M.: Effect of hydrocortisone on response of lymphocytes to stimulation by sodium periodate. Clin Immunol Immunopath *5*, 177 (1976)
223. Segel, G. B., Lukacher, A., Gordon, B. R., Lichtman, M. A.: Glucocorticoid suppression of human lymphocyte DNA synthesis: Influence of phytohemagglutinin concentration. J Lab Clin Med *95*, 624 (1980)
224. Taetle, R., Guittard, J. P.: Modulation of leukaemia blast colony growth by steroid hormones. Br J Haematol *50*, 247 (1982)
225. Winkelstein, A.: The effect of cyclosporin and hydrocortisone on human T-lymphocyte colony formation. Cell Immunol *86*, 413 (1984)
226. Galanaud, P., Crevon, M. C., Emilie, D., Abella, A.: Effect of hydrocortisone on the *in vitro* human antibody response: Interaction with Monocytes and Prostaglandins. Clin Immunol Immunopath *29*, 403 (1983)
227. Ambrose, C. T.: The essential role of corticosteroids in the induction of the immune response

in vitro. In: Hormones and the Immune Response (ed.). Wolstenholme, G. E., Knight, J.; Ciba Foundation Study Group No. 36, pub.: J. A. Churchill, London. p 100 (1970)
228. Dupont, E., Schandene, L., Devos, R., Lambermont, M., Wybran, J.: Depletion of lymphocytes with membrane markers of helper phenotype: A feature of acute and chronic druginduced immunosuppression. Clin Exp Immunol *51*, 345 (1983)
229. Charpenter, B., Lang, P., Martin, B., Fries, D.: Evidence for a suppressor cell system in human kidney allograft tolerance. Transplant Proc *13*, 90 (1981)
230. Liburd, E., Pazderka, V., Kovithavongs, T., Dossetor, J. B.: Evidence for suppressor cells, and reduced CML induction by the donor in transplant patients. Transplant Proc *10*, 557 (1978)
231. Thomas, J., Thomas, F., Lee, H. M.: Why do HLA-non-identical renal allografts survive 10 years or more? Transplant Proc *9*, 85 (1977)
232. Bell, P. A., Munck, A.: Steroid-binding properties and stabilization of cytoplasmic glucocorticoid receptors from rat thymus cells. Biochem J *136*, 97 (1973)
233. Picard, F., Homo, F., Duval, D.: Effect of glucocorticoids on cholesterol synthesis in isolated mouse thymocytes. J Ster Biochem *12*, 253 (1980)
234. Whitelaw, M. J.: Physiological reaction to pituitary adrenocorticotropic hormone in severe burns. J Am Med Assoc *195*, 85 (1951)
235. Medawer, P. P., Sparrow, E. M.: Effect of adrenocortical hormones, adrenocorticotropic hormone and pregnancy on skin transplantation immunity. J Endo *14*, 240 (1956)
236. Sparrow, E. M.: Effect of cortisone, alcohol and ACTH on skin homografts in guinea pigs. J Endo *11*, 57 (1954)
237. Ellison, E. H., Martin, B. C., Williams, R. D., Chatworthy, H. W., Hanewi, G., Zollinger, R. M.: Adrenal cortical hormone and homografting. Ann Surg *134*, 495 (1951)
238. Krohn, P. L.: Effect of steroid hormones on survival of skin grafts in the rabbit. J Endo *11*, 78 (1954)
239. Perky, L., Jacob, S.: Effect of ACTH and cortisone on homologous kidney transplant. Proc Soc Exp Bio Med *77*, 66 (1951)
240. Comsa, J., Leonhardt, H., Schwarz, J. A.: Influence of the thymus-corticotropin-growth hormone interaction on the rejection of skin allografts in the rat. Ann NY Acad Sci *249*, 387 (1975)
241. Dameshek, W., Rosenthal, M. C., Schwartz, L.: Treatment of acquired hemolytic anemia with ACTH. N Eng J Med *244*, 117 (1950)
242. Bjoernboe, M.: Serum protein during immunization. Acta Path Microbio Scand *20*, 221 (1943)
243. Bjoernboe, M., Fischell, E. F., Stoerk, H. C.: Effect of ACTH and cortisone on concentration of circulating antibodies. J Exp Med *93*, 37 (1951)
244. Hayes, S. P., Dougherty, T. F.: Effect of ACTH and cortisone on antibody synthesis and rate of disappearance of antigen. Fed Proc *11*, 67 (1952)
245. Moechlin, S., Baguerra, R., Baguerra, T.: Influence of ACTH and cortisone on experimental antibody production in rabbits. Bull Schweiz Akad Med Wiss *8*, 153 (1953)
246. Newson, S. E., Darrach, M.: Effect of corticotropin and corticosteroid on the production of hemolytic anntibodies in the mouse. Can J Biochem Physiol *32*, 372 (1954)
247. Kass, E. H., Kendrick, M. L., Finland, M.: Effect of corticosterone, hydrocortisone and corticotropin on the production of antibodies in rabbits. J Exp Med *102*, 767 (1955)
248. Elliott, E. V., Sinclair, N. R.: Effect of cortisone acetatye on 19s and 7s haemolysin antibody. A time course study. Immunol *15*, 643 (1968)
249. Mantzouranis, E., Borel, Y.: Different effects of cortisone on the humoral immune response to T-independent antigens. Cell Immunol *43*, 202 (1979)
250. Claman, H. N., Moorehead, J. W., Benner, W. H.: Corticosteroids and lymphoid cells *in vitro*. I. Hydrocortisone lysis of human, guinea pig, and mouse thymus cells. J Lab Clin Med *78*, 499 (1971)
251. Blomgren, H., Anderson, B.: Characterization of the immunocompetent cells in mouse thymus: Cell population changes during cortisone-induced atrophy and subsequent regeneration. Cell Immunol *11*, 545 (1971)
252. Hochman, P. S., Cudkowicz, G.: Different sensitivities to hydrocortisone of natural killer cell activity and by hybrid resistance to parental marrow grafts. J Immunol *119*, 2013 (1977)
253. Lotzova, E., Savary, C. A.: Parallelism between the effect of cortisone acetate in hybrid resistance and natural killing. Exp Hematol *9*, 766 (1981)

254. Thompson, J., Van Furth, R.: The effect of glucocorticosteroids on the kinetics of mononuclear phagocytes. J Exp Med *131*, 429 (1970)
255. Von den Brock, A. A., Keuning, F. J., Soeharto, R., Prop, N.: Immune suppression and histophysiology of immune response. Virchows Arch [Cell Path] *3*, 43 (1983)
256. Ernstrom, V.: Hormonal influences on thymic release of lymphocytes into the blood. In: Hormones and the Immune Response (ed.). Wolstenholme, G. E. W., Knight, J.; Ciba Foundation Study Group No. 36, Pub.: J. A. Churchill, London; p 53 (1970)
257. Snyder, D. S., Unane, E. R.: Corticosteroids inhibit murine macrophage Ia expression and interleukin 1 production. J Immunol *129*, 1803 (1982)
258. Gillis, S., Crabtree, G. R., Smith, K.: Glucocorticoidinduced inhibition of T cell growth factor production. I. The Effect of Mitogen-induced lymphocyte proliferation. J Immunol *123*, 1624 (1979)
259. Kelso, A., Munck, H.: Glucorticoid inhibition of lymphokine secretion by alloreactive T-lymphocyte clones. J Immunol *133*, 784 (1984)
260. Besedovsky, H. O., Rey, A. D., Sorken, E., Lotz, W., Schwulera, U.: Lymphoid cells produce an immunoregulatory glucocorticoid increasing factor (GIF) acting through the pituitary gland. Clin Exp Immunol *59*, 622 (1985)
261. Nemeroff, C. B., Widerlov, E., Bissette, G., Wallens, H., Karlsson, K., Eklund, K., Kilts, C. D., Loosen, P. T., Vale, W.: Elevated concentrations of CSF corticotropin-releasing factor-like immuno reactivity in depressed patients. Science *226*, 1342 (1984)
262. Bartrop, R. W., Lazarus, L., Luckhurst, E., Kiloh, L. G.: Depressed lymphocyte function after bereavement. Lancet, *April 16*, 834 (1977)
263. Wolfe, J. H. N., Wu, A. V. O., O'Conner, N. E., Saparoschetz, I., Mannick, J. A.: Anergy, immunosuppressive serum, and impaired lymphocyte blastogenesis in burn patients. Arch Surg *117*, 1266 (1982)
264. Watson, R. R., Chien, G., Chung, C.: Thymosin treatment: serum corticosterone and lymphocyte mitogenesis in moderately and severely protein-malnourished mice. J Nutr *113*, 483 (1983)
265. Sapolsky, R. M., Donnelly, T. M.: Vulnerability to stress-induced tumor growth increases with age in rats: role of glucocorticoids. Endocrinol *117*, 662 (1985)
266. Krieger, D.: Cushing's Syndrome. Springer-Verlag, Berlin (1982)
267. Galland, R. B., Heine, K. J., Polk, HK. C.: Nonspecific stimulation of host defenses against bacterial challenge in immunosuppressed mice. Arch Surg *118*, 333 (1983)
268. Blackwood, L. L., Pennington, J. E.: Dose-dependent effect of glucocorticoids on pulmonary defenses in a steroid-resistant host. Am Rev Respir Dis *126*, 1045 (1982)
269. Genovesi, E. V., Livnat, D., Collins, J. J.: Immune therapy of murine leukemia. VII. Efficacy of passive serum therapy of friend leukemia virus-induced disease in immunocompromised mice. J Nat Can Inst *70*, 311 (1983)
270. Stevens, W., Colessides, C., Dougherty, T.: Effects of cortisol on the incorporation of thymidine-2-^{14}C into nucleic acids and lymphatic tissue from adrenalectomized CBA mice. Endocrinol *76*, 1100 (1965)
271. Stevens, W., Colessides, C., Dougherty, T.: A time study on the effect of cortisol on the incorporation of thymidine-2-^{14}C into nucleic acids of mouse lymphatics. Endocrinology *78*, 600 (1966)
272. Kidson, C.: Cortisol in the regulation of RNA and protein synthesis. Nature *213*, 779 (1967)
273. Beck, J., Browning, M.: Immunosuppression wich glucocorticoid — a possible immunological explanation for interpatient variation and sensitivity: Discussion paper. J Royal Soc Med *76*, 473 (1983)
274. Crabtree, G., Gillis, S., Smith, K., Munck, A.: Glucocorticoids and immune response. Arth Rheum *22*, 1246 (1979)
275. Zweiman, B., Atkins, P., Bedard, P., Flaschen, S., Lisak, R.: Corticosteroid effects on circulating lymphocyte subset levels in normal humans. J Clin Immunol *4*, 151 (1984)
276. Grieco, M.: The role of corticosteroid therapy in infection. Hosp Pract *19*, 131 (1984)
277. MacGregor, R., Spagnuolo, P., Lentner, A.: Inhibition of granulocyte adherence by ethanol, prednisone, and aspirin measured with an assay system. N Eng J Med *291*, 642 (1974)
278. Allen, N., Kissel, P., Pietrasiuk, D., Perlow, M.: Myasthenia gravis in monozygotic twins. Arch Neurol *41*, 994 (1984)

279. Berrih, S., Safar, D., Levasseur, P., Gaud, C., Bach, J.: The *in vivo* effects of corticosteroids on thymocyte subsets in myasthenia gravis. J Clin Immunol *4*, 92 (1984)
280. Nagy, E., Berczi, I.: Immunodeficiency in hypophysectomized rats. Acta Endocrinol *89*, 530 (1978)
281. Berczi, I., Nagy, E., Kovacs, K., Horvath, E.: Regulation of humoral immunity in rats by pituitary hormones. Acta Endocrinol *98*, 506 (1981)
282. Nagy, E., Berczi, I., Friesen, H. G.: Regulation of immunity in rats by lactogenic and growth hormones. Acta Endocrinol *102*, 351 (1983)
283. Nagy, E., Berczi, I.: Prolactin and contact sensitivity. Allergy *36*, 429 (1981)
284. Berczi, I., Nagy, E., Asa, S. L., Kovacs, K.: Pituitary hormones and contact sensitivity in rats. Allergy *38*, 325 (1983)
285. Nagy, E., Friesen, H. G., Sehon, A. H., Berczi, I.: Immunomodulation in rats by transplantable anterior pituitary tumors. Endocrinol *116*, 1117 (1985)
286. Cross, R. J., Brooks, W. H., Roszman, T. L., Markesbery, W. R.: Hypothalamic-immune interactions. Effects of hypophysectomy on neuroimmunomodulation. J Neurology Sci *53*, 557 (1982)
287. Harrison, D. E., Archer, J. R., Astle, C. M.: The effect of hypophysectomy on thymic aging in mice. J Immunol *129*, 2673 (1982)
288. Scott, M., Bolla, R.: Age-related changes in immune function of rats and the effect of long-term hypophysectomy. Mech Age Develop *11*, 127 (1979)
289. Makinodan, T.: Control of immunologic abnormalities associated with aging. Mech Age Develop *9*, 7 (1979)
290. Builder, G. E., Denckla, W. D.: Restoration of ability to reject xenografts and clear carbon after hypophysectomy of adult rats. Mech Age Develop *6*, 153 1977)
291. Parker, R. J., Bekowitz, B. A., Lee, C. H., Denckla, W. D.: Vascular relaxation, aging and thyroid hormones. Mech Age Develop *8*, 397 (1978)
292. Bolla, R., Denckla, D.: Effect of hypophysectomy on liver nuclear ribonucleic acid synthesis in aging rats. Biochem J *184*, 669 (1979)
293. Denckla, W. D.: Interactions between age and the neuroendocrine and immune systems. Fed Proc *37*, 1263 (1978)
294. Pandian, M. R., Talwar, G. P.: Effect of growth hormone on the metabolism of thymus and on the immune response against sheep erythrocytes. J Exp Med *134*, 1095 (1971)
295. Talwar, G. P., Hanjan, S. N. S., Kidwai, Z., Gupta, P. D., Mehrotra, N. N., Saxena, R., Bhattarai, Q.: Growth hormone action on thymus and lymphoid cells. Proc IIIrd Internat Symp Milan, Sept. 17–20, 1975; Ed: Pecile, A., Muller, E. E.; Pub: Exerpta Medica, Amsterdam; American Elsevier Pub Co, NY, pp 104–115 (1976)
296. Gisler, R. H., Schenkel-Hulliger, L.: Hormonal regulation of the immune response. II. Influence of pituitary and adrenal activity on immune responsiveness *in vitro*. Cell Immunol *2*, 646 (1971)
297. Comsa, J., Schwarz, J. A., Neu, H.: Interaction between thymic hormone and hypophyseal growth hormone on production of precipitating antibodies in the rat. Immunol Commun *3*, 11 (1974)
298. Arrenbrecht, S., Sorkin, E.: Growth hormone-induced T-cell differentiation. Eur J Immunol *3*, 601 (1973)
299. Pierpaoli, W., Sorkin, E.: A study on anti-pituitary serum. Immunol *16*, 311 (1969)
300. Snow, C. E., Feldbush, T. L., Oaks, J. A.: The effect of growth hormone and insulin upon MLR responses and the generation of cytotoxic lymphocytes. J Immunol *126*, 161 (1981)
301. Astaldi, A., Yalcin, B., Meardi, G., Burgio, G. R., Merolla, R., Astaldi, G.: Effect of growth hormone on lymphocyte transformation in cell culture. Blut Banc XXVI, 74 (1973)
302. Kiess, W., Holtmann, H., Butenandt, O., Eife, R.: Modulation of lymphoproliferation by human growth hormone. Eur J Pediatr *140*, 47 (1983)
303. Astaldi, G., Burgio, G. R., Astaldi, A., Yalcin, B., Meardi, G., Gatti, G.: Growth hormone and lymphocyte activation. Lancet *Sept. 30*, 709 (1972)
304. Mercola, K. E., Cline, M. J., Golde, D. W.: Growth hormone stimulation of normal and leukemic human T-lymphocyte proliferation *in vitro*. Blood *58*, 337 (1981)
305. Vanderschueren-Lodeweyckk, M., Staf, B., Eggermont, E., Eeckels, R.: Growth Hormone and lymphocyte transformation. Lancet *Feb. 24*, 441 (1973)
306. Pierpaoli, W., Fabris, N., Sorkin, E.: Developmental hormones and immunological maturation.

Hormones and the Immune Response, Ciba Foundation Study Group No. 36; Ed: Wolstenholme, G. E., Knight, J.; Pub: J. A. Churchilll, London, pp 126–153 (1970)
307. Billingham, R. E.: The biology of graft-versus-host reactions. Harvey Lect *62*, 21 (1967)
308. Pierpaoli, W., Sorkin, E.: Effect of growth hormone and anti-growth hormone serum on the lymphatic tissue and the immune response. Antibiotica Chemothera *15*, 122 (1969)
309. Duquesnoy, R. J., Ahrens, R. C.: Increased responsiveness to phytochemagglutinin and graft-versus-host reactivity of thymus cells from Snell-Bagg Dwarf Mice. J Immunol *110*, 578 (1973)
310. Dumont, F., Robert, F., Bischoff, P.: T- and B-lymphocytes in pituitary dwarf Snell-Bagg Mice. Immunol *38*, 23 (1979)
311. Pierpaoli, W., Baroni, C., Fabris, N., Sorkin, E.: Hormones and immunological capacity. II. Reconstitution of antibody production in hormonally deficient mice by somatotropic hormone, thyrotropic hormone and thyroxin. Immunol *16*, 217 (1969)
312. Baroni, C. D., Scelsi, R., Mingazzini, P. L., Cavallero, A., Uccini, S.: Delayed hypersensitivity in the hereditary pituitary dwarf Snell/Bagg mouse. Nature New Biol *237*, 219 (1972)
313. Baroni, C. D., Fabris, N., Bertoli, G.: Effects of hormones on development and function of lymphoid tissues. Synergistic action of thyroxin and somatotropic hormone in pituitary dwarf mice. Immunol *17*, 303 (1969)
314. Roth, J. A., Lomax, L. G., Altszuler, N., Hampshire, J., Kaeberle, M. L., Shelton, M., Draper, D. D., Ledet, A. E.: Thymic abnormalities and growth hormone deficiency in dogs. Am J Vet Res *41*, 1256 (1980)
315. Roth, J. A., Kaeberle. M. L., Grier, R. L., Hopper, J. G., Spiegel, H. E., McAllister, H. A.: Improvement in clinical condition and thymus morphologic features associated with growth hormone treatment of immunodeficient dwarf dogs. Am J Vet Res *45*, 1151 (1984)
316. Thierist-Prevost, G., Schumpff, R-M, Sharif, A.: A hormonally-controlled serum factor stimulating the thymidine uptake into lectin-activated lymphocytes. Acta Endocrinol *98*, 358 (1981)
317. Bajoruunas, D., Brockman, R., Cunningham-Rundles, S., Sonenberg, M.: Growth hormone modulation of human immune parameters. Endo Soc., 64th Annual Meeting, Abst. *96*, 103 (1982)
318. Rogers, P. C., Komp, D., Rogol, A., Sabio, H.: Possible effects of growth hormone on development of acute lymphoblastic leukaemia. Lancet *Aug. 27*, 434 (1977)
319. Ammann, A. J., Duquesnoy, R. J., Good, R. A.: Endocrinological studies in ataxia, telangiectasia and other immunological deficiency diseases. Clin Exp Immunol *6*, 587 (1970)
320. Abbassi, V., Bellanti, J. A.: Humoral and cell-mediated immunity in growth hormone-deficient children: Effect of therapy with human growth hormone. Ped Res *19*, 299 (1985)
321. Sotowska-Brochocka, J., Rosolowska-Huszcz, D., Skwarlo-Sonta, K., Gajewska, A.: Effect of exogeneous prolactin on immunity in chickens. Res Vet Sci *37*, 123 (1984)
322. Singh, U., Owen, J. J. T.: Studies on the maturation of thymus stem cells. The effects of catecholamines, histamine and peptide hormones on the expression of T-cell alloantigens. Eur J Immunol *6*, 59 (1976)
323. Karmali, R. A., Lauder, I., Horrobin, D. F.: Prolactin and immune response. Lancet *July 13*, 106 (1974)
324. Pierpaoli, W., Kopp, H. G., Bianchi, E.: Interdependence of thymic and neuroendocrine functions in ontogeny. Clin Exp Immunol *24*, 501 (1976)
325. Giguere, V., Meunier, H., Veilleux, R., Labrie, F.: Direct effects of sex steroids on prolactin release at the anterior pituitary level: Interactions with dopamine, thyrotropin-releasing hormone, and isobutylmethylxanthine. Endocrinol *111*, 857 (1982)
326. Labrie, F., Beaulieu, M., Caron, M. G., Raymond, V.: The adenohypophyseal dopamine receptor: specificity and modulation of its activity by estradiol. In: Robyn, C., Harter, M. (ed.). Progress in Prolactin Physiology and Pathology. Elsevier/North-Holland, Amsterdam, p. 121 (1978)
327. Raymond, V., Beaulieu, M., Labrie, F., Boissier, J. R.: Potent antidopaminergic activity of estradiol at the pituitary level on prolactin release. Science *200*, 1173 (1978)
328. Sharp, S. E., Phares, C. K., Heidrick, M. L.: Immunological aspects associated with suppression of hormone levels in rats infected with plerocercoids of Spirometra mansonoides (cestoda). J Parasital *68*, 993 (1982)
329. Bilder, G. E., Denckla, W. D.: Restoration of ability to reject xenografts and clear carbon after hypophysectomy of adult rats. Mech Age Develop *6*, 153 (1977)
330. Pacini, F., Nakamura, H., DeGroot, L. J.: Effect of hypo- and hyperthyroidism on the balance between helper and suppressor T-cells in rats. Acta Endocrinol *103*, 528 (1983)

331. Balazs, C. S., Farid, N. R.: Effect of triiodothyronine on the short-lived and concanavalin-A generated suppressor T-cell functions. Clin Invest Med *7*, 157 (1984)
332. Kidd, A., Okita, N., Row, V. V., Volpe, R.: Immunologic aspects of Graves and Hashimoto's diseases. Metab *29*, 80 (1980)
333. Burman, K. D., Baker, J. R.: Immune mechanisms in Graves disease. Endocrine Rev *6*, 193 (1985)
334. Makinen, T., Wagner, G., Apter, L., VonWillebrand, E., Pekonen, F.: Evidence that the TSH receptor acts as a mitogenic antigen in Graves disease. Nature *275*, 314 (1978)
335. Wenzel, B., Kotulla, P., Wenzel, K. W., Finke, R., Schleusener, H.: Mitogenic response of peripheral blood lymphocytes from patients with Graves' disease incubated with solubilized thyroid cell membranes containing TSH receptor and with thyroglobulin. Immunobiol *160*, 302 (1981)
336. Rebar, R. W., Morandini, I. C., Silva de Sa, M. F., Erickson, G. F., Petze, J. E.: The importance of the thymus gland for normal reproductive function in mice. In: Schwartz, N. B., Hunzikker-Dunn, M. (eds.). Dynamics of Ovarian Function. Raven Pres, New York, p 285 (1981)
337. Rebar, R. W., Miyaka, A., Erickson, G. F., Low, T. L. K., Goldstein, A. L.: The influence of the thymus gland on reproductive function: A hypothalamic site of action. In: Greenwald, G. S., Terranova, P. F. (eds.). Factors Regulating Ovarian Function. Raven Press, New York, p 465 (1983)
338. Michael, S. D., Taguchi, O., Nisizuka, Y., McClure, J. E., Goldstein, A. L., Barkley, M. S.: The effects of neonatal thymectomy on early follicular loss and circulating levels of corticosterone, progesterone, estradiol and thymosin. In: Schwartz, N. V., Hunzicker-Dunn, M. (eds.). Dynamics of Ovarian Function. Raven Press, New York, p 279 (1981)
339. Michael, S. D., Taguchi, O., Nishizuka, Y.: Effect of neonatal thymectomy on ovarian development and plasma LH, FSH, GH and PRL in the mouse. Biol Reprod *22*, 343 (1980)
340. Michael, S. D.: The role of the endocrine thymus in female reproduction. Arth Rheum *22*, 1241 (1981)
341. Hattori, M., Brandon, M. R.: Thymus and the endocrine system: Ovarian dysgenesis in neonatally thymectomied rats. J Endocrinol *83*, 101 (1983)
342. Michael, S. D.: Interactions of the thymus and the ovary. In: Greenwald, G. S., Terranova, P. F. (eds.). Factors Regulating Ovarian Function. Raven Press, New York, p 445 (1983)
343. Bukovsky, A., Presl, J.: Ovarian function and the immune system. Med Hypoth *5*, 415 (1979)
344. Espey, L. L.: Ovulation as an inflammatory reaction — a hypothesis. Biol Repro *22*, 73 (1980)
345. Farooki, R.: Atresia: an hypothesis. In: Schwartz, N. B., Hunzicker-Dunn, M. (eds.). Dynamics of Ovarian Function. Raven Press, NYI p 13 (1981)
346. Seemayer, T., Laroche, A., Russo, P., Maoebranche, R., Arnoux, E., Guerin, J., Pierre, G., Dupuy, J., Gartner, J., Lapp, W., Spira, T., Lelie, R.: Precocious thymus involution manifest by epithelial injury in the ascquired immune deficiency syndrome. Human Path *15*, 469 (1984)
347. Tsuchiya, M.: Immunological abnormalities involving the thymus in ulcerative colitis and therapeutic effects of thymectomy. Gastroenterologia Japon *19*, 232 (1984)
348. Barlas, N., Mutchnick, M., Grant, G., Trainin, N.: The effect of thymic humoral factor on intracellular lymphocyte cyclic AMP in alcoholic liver disease. Thymus *5*, 433 (1983)
349. Stiehm, E.: Immundeficiency — an overview. Chest *86*D, 20S (1984)
350. Rosenow, E., Hurley, B.: Disorders of the thymus — a review. Arch Internal Med *144*, 763 (1984)
351. Monden, Y., Nakahar, K., Kagotani, K., Fujii, Y., Nanjo, S. A., Kawashima, Y.: Effects of preoperative duration of symptoms on patients with myasthenia gravis. Annals Thorac Surg *38*, 287 (1984)
352. Fabris, N., Amadio, L., Licastro, F., Mocchegiani, E., Zannotti, M., Franceschi, C., Thymic hormone deficiency in normal aging and Downs syndrome — Is there a primary failure of the thymus? Lancet *1*, 983 (1984)
353. Baroini, C., Avaltieri, M., Stoppacciaro, A., Ruco, L., Uccini, S., Ricci, C.: The human thymus in aging: Histologic involution paralleled by increased mitogen response by enrichment of OKT3 lymphocytes. Immunol *50*, 519 (1983)
354. Beatty, D., Handzel, Z., Pecht, M., Ryder, C., Hughes, J., McCabe, K., Trainin, N.: A controlled trial of treatment of acquired immune deficiency in severe measles with thymic humoral factor. Clin Exp Immunol *56*, 479 (1984)

355. Mills, J.: Transmission processes between clock and manifestation. In: Biological Aspects of Circadian Rhythms, ed: Mills, J. N., pub: Plenum Press, NY, p 28–84 (1973)
356. Fuller, R., Diller, E.: Diurnal variation of liver glycogen and plasma free fatty acids in rats fed ad libitum or single daily meal. Metabol *19*, 226 (1970)
357. MacVerry, P., Kim, K.: Diurnal rhythms of rat liver glycogen synthetase. Biochem Biophys Res Commun *46*, 1242 (1972)
358. Suttie, J. W.: Effect of dietary fluoride on the pattern of food intake in rat and the development of a programmed pellet dispenser. J Nutr *96*, 529 (1968)
359. Morris, H. G., Jorgensen, J. R.: Circadian pattern of plasma GH concentration in children. Clin Res *16*, 248 (1968)
360. Freinkel, N., Mager, M., Vinnick, L.: Cyclicity in the inter GH relationships between plasma insulin and glucose during starvation in normal young men. J Lab Clin Med *71*, 171 (1968)
361. Hellamn, B., Hellerstrom, C.: Diurnal changes in the function of the pancreatic islets of rats as indicated by nuclear size in the islet cells. Acta Endocrinol *31*, 267 (1959)
362. Shimazu, T., Amakawa, A.: Regulation of glycogen metabolism in liver by autonomic nervous system. II. Neural control of glycogenolytic enzymes. Biochem Biophys Acta *165*, 335 (1968)
363. Barbason, H., Van Cantfort, J.: Nyctohemeral rhythms in the liver. In: Progress in Liver Diseases, Vol. V, p 136 (1976)
364. Jaffe, J. J.: Diurnal mitotic periodicity in regenerating rat liver. Anat Rec *120*, 935 (1954)
365. Fabrikant, J.: The kinetics of cellular proliferation in regenerating liver. J Cell Biol *36*, 551 (1968)
366. Heine, W. D., Stocker, E., Heine, H. D.: Tageszeitliche Rhythmen der Zellproliferation in der kompensatorisch regenerierenden Niere nach unilateraler Nephrektomie. Virchows Arch (Zellpathol) *9*, 75 (1971)
367. Reiter, R. J.: Circannual reproductive rhythm in mammals related to photoperiod and pineal function. A review. Chronobiologia *1*, 365 (1974)
368. Hoffman, K.: Photoperiodic mechanisms in hamsters: The participation of the pineal gland. In: Environmental Endocrinology, ed: Assenmacher, I., Farner, D. S.; Pub: Springer-Verlag, Berlin, p 94 (1978)
369. Hoffmann, J. C., Kordon, C., Benoit, J.: Effect of different photoperiods and blinding on ovarian and testicular functions in normal and testosterone treated rats. Gen Comp Endocrinol *10*, 109 (1968)
370. Reiter, R. J., Hoffmann, J. C., Rubin, P. H.: Pineal gland: Influence on gonads of male rats treated with androgen three days after birth. Science *160*, 420 (1968)
371. Vanecek, J., Illnerova, H.: Effect of photoperiod on the growth of reproductive organs and on pineal N-acetyltransferase rhythm in male rats treated neonatally with testosterone propionate. Biol Repro *27*, 517 (1982)
372. Tetsuo, M., Perlow, M. J., Mishkin, M., Markey, S. P.: Light exposure reduces and pinealectomy virtually stops urinary excretion of 6-hydroxymelatonin by Rhesus Monkeys. Endocrinol *110*, 997 (1982)
373. Martin, J. E., McKeel, D. W., Sattler, C.: Melatonin directly inhibits rat gonadotroph cells. Endocrinol *110*, 1079 (1982)
374. Pownall, R., Knapp, M. S.: Immune responses have rhythms: Are they important? Cell Memb Biol *8*, VII (1980)
375. Pownall, R., Knapp, M. S.: Circadian Rhythmicity of delayed hypersensitivity to oxazolone in the rat. Clin Sci *54*, 447 (1978)
376. Fernandes, G., Halberg, F., Yunis, E. J., Good, R. A.: Circadian rhythmic plaque-forming cell response of spleens from mice immunized with SRBC. J Immunol *117*, 962 (1976)
377. McGilles, J. P., Hall, N. R., Goldstein, A. L.: Circadian rhythm of thymosin, in normal and thymectomized mice. J Immunol *131*, 148 (1983)
378. Bershol, J. F., McClure, J. E., Yamamoto, W. S., Goldstein, A. L.: Evidence for a circadian rhythm of thymosin$_1$, in humans. Personal communication
379. Mochizuki, M., Charley, A., Kuwabara, T., Nussenblatt, R., Gery, I.: Involvement of the pineal gland in rats with experimental autoimmune uveitis. Investigative Ophthalmology and Visual Science *24*, 1333 (1983)
380. Williams, G., Ghanadian, R., Papadopoulos, A. S., Costro, J. E.: Hormonal environment of immunosuppressed mice. Br J Cancer *37*, 123 (1978)
381. Fabris, N., Pierpaoli, W., Sorkin, E.: Hormones and the immunological capacity. III. The

immunodeficiency disease of the hypopituitary Snell-Bagg dwarf mouse. Clin Exp Immunol *9*, 209 (1971)

382. Rebar, R. W., Miyaka, A., Low, T. L. K., Goldstein, A. A.: Thymosin stimulates secretion of luteinizing hormonereleasing factor. Science *214*, 669 (1981)
383. Hall, N. R., McGillis, J. P., Spangelo, B. L., Goldstein, A. L.: Evidence that thymosins and other biological response modifiers can function as neuroactive immunotransmitters. J Immunol *135*, 806S (1985)
384. Rebar, R. W., Morandini, I. C., Petze, J. E., Erickson, G. F.: Hormonal basis of reproductive defects in athymic mice: reduced gonadotropin and testosterone in males. Biol Repro *27*, 1267 (1982)
385. Rebar, R. W., Morandini, I. C., Erickson, G. F., Petze, J. E.: The hormonal basis of reproductive defects in a thymic mice: diminished gonadotropin concentrations in prepubertal females. Endocrinol *108*, 120 (1981)
386. Besedovsky, H. O., Sorkin, E.: Thymus involvement in female sexual maturation. Nature *249*, 356 (1974)
387. Allen, L. S., McClure, J. E., Goldstein, A. L., Barkley, M. S., Michaell, S. D.: Estrogen and thymic hormone interactions in the female mouse. J Repro Immunol *6*, 25 (1983)
388. Rivier, C., Vale, W.: Influence of corticotropin-releasing factor on reproductive functions in the rat. Endocrinol *114*, 914 (1984)
389. Ringstrom, S. J., Schwartz, N. B.: Examination of prolactin and pituitary-adrenal axis components as intervening variables in the adrenelectomy-induced inhibition of gonadotropin response in castration. Endocrinol *114*, 880 (1984)
390. Hall, N. R., Goldstein, A. L.: Neurotransmitters and the immune system. In: Psychoneuroimmunology, Ed: Ader, R.; Pub: Academic Press, NY, p 521 (1981)
391. Besedovsky, H., Sorkin, E.: Network of immune-neuroendocrine interactions. Clin Exp Immunol *27*, 1 (1972)
392. Marx, J. L.: The immune system "belongs in the body." Science *227*, 1190 (1985)
393. Dann, J. A., Wachtel, S. S., Rubin, A. L.: Possible involvement of the central nervous system in graft rejection. Transplan *27*, 223 (1979)
394. Pierpaoli, W., Kopp, H. G., Muller, J., Keller, M.: Interdependence between neuroendocrine programming and the generation of immune recognition in ontogeny. Cell Immunol *29*, 16 (1977)
395. Bovbjerg, D., Cohen, N., Ader, R.: The central nervous system and learning: a strategy for immune regulation. Immunol Today *3*, 287 (1982)

Malaria Vaccine

W. Trager, M. E. Perkins, and H. N. Lanners*

The Rockefeller University, 1230 York Avenue New York, New York 10021, U.S.A.

As a result of the development and application during the last 10 years of culture methods and the methods of monoclonal antibody production and of recombinant DNA technology, there are now available for testing a number of potential malaria vaccines, particularly against *Plasmodium falciparum*. The sporozoite vaccines are directed against the circumsporozoite protein and include synthetic peptides containing several repeats of the immunodominant tetrapeptide as well as larger portions of the antigen cloned and expressed in *Escherichia coli*. The erythrocytic stages present a number of target antigens. Of special interest are proteins identified from the surface and rhoptries of merozoites, several of which have been cloned and expressed in *E. coli* and at least one of which has given protective immunity in *Saimiri* monkeys. With sporozoite vaccines now under trial in human volunteers and with several potential merozoite vaccines being tested in experimental monkeys the time for field trials is rapidly approaching. In addition several gamete antigens have been isolated and may prove effective for the induction of transmission-blocking immunity.

* Present address: Department of Tropical Medicine, Tulane University Medical Center, New Orleans, Louisiana 70112

1 Introduction

Malaria is a disease of long duration and chronicity. Typical infections with *Plasmodium vivax* or *P. ovale* last 2 to 3 years, with periodic remissions and relapses. *P. malariae* may persist as a latent inapparent infection up to 50 years. Even with *P. falciparum*, the most highly pathogenic species of human malaria, immunity develops only slowly [1]. Under natural conditions in a holoendemic region where exposure to reinfection is frequent and sustained, children that survive their initial infections show an enlarged spleen and are likely to continue to show parasites until puberty, or even beyond. In such a region adults do not have a markedly enlarged spleen, rarely show parasites and are rarely ill with malaria. This acquired immunity is effective mainly against the local strains of falciparum malaria and fades rapidly if the individual lives for some months in a non-malarious region. Nevertheless, if such an immunity could be induced earlier by vaccination, and especially if it could be induced in young children, many lives would be saved and much illness prevented. An effective vaccine would also serve as an additional tool which, combined with mosquito control measures and appropriate chemotherapy, might greatly reduce the incidence of malaria. Clearly a vaccine could also be useful for the protection of short term visitors to malarious regions. Such protection is becoming increasingly difficult to provide as drugresistant strains of *P. falciparum* continue to spread [2].

Acquired immunity to malaria depends on both humoral antibodies and cell-mediated mechanisms. This has been clearly shown for human malaria as well as in a wide variety of experimental model systems using species of malarial parasites infective to convenient laboratory hosts: avian malaria in chickens, rodent malaria in mice, and simian malaria in rhesus monkeys [3-11]. These experimental studies showed furthermore the existence of stage-specific antigens and stage-specific immunity. Animals immunized only with sporozoites, the infective forms inoculated by mosquitoes, were fully susceptible to infection by the erythrocytic stages of the same species. Conversely, animals made immune by exposure only to the erythrocytic stages would still support the development of sporozoites to preerythrocytic forms. This led to the concept of stage-specific vaccines: an anti-sporozoite vaccine and an anti-erythrocytic stage vaccine, more briefly known as the sporozoite vaccine and the merozoite vaccine. In addition there developed the possibility of an anti-gamete or transmission-blocking vaccine; antibodies to gametes taken up with its bloodmeal by a mosquito inactivate the gametes in the mosquito's midgut thereby preventing its infection. Until ten years ago there was no practical way to produce enough antigen for any of these potential vaccines. No stage of any malaria parasite could be cultured *in vitro* and there was no experimental animal that could be used to produce sufficient amounts of human malaria parasites. Then came three almost simultaneous developments that now make possible the imminent trial in humans of the first potential anti-malaria vaccines:

(1) Continuous culture of *P. falciparum* in vitro [12,13]. This provides a convenient laboratory source of material for preparation and fractionation of antigen in amounts sufficient for pilot trials of merozoite vaccines in experimental animals. It also makes possible the separation and identification of strains and clones of *P. falciparum* [14] from different geographic regions, and the comparative study of their genomes [15].

The production of gametocytes in the cultures furthermore makes possible the study of gamete antigens [16] and also permits the ready infection of mosquitoes in the laboratory to provide sporozoites for studies related to a sporozoite vaccine.

(2) Monoclonal antibodies [17]. This powerful technique enables the identification and localization of specific antigens.

(3) Recombinant DNA technology. This permits sequencing of genes for specific antigens, in this way providing information on the structure of immunodominant epitopes, and also permits the ultimate large scale production of the antigen or of sequences constituting the identified epitopes.

2 Sporozoite Vaccine

Without these last two developments a sporozoite vaccine would have been completely impractical. Through their elegant application largely by R. S. Nussenzweig and her colleagues, a sporozoite vaccine is about to undergo preliminary trials in humans. Immunization with inactivated sporozoites was first shown for *P. gallinaceum* in chickens [18], but little further work was done until the *P. berghei*-mouse-*Anopheles stephensi* system was developed. In this model sporozoites of *P. berghei* appropriately treated with X-rays to render them noninfective though still antigenic would induce in mice a strong immunity to challenge with live sporozoites [19]. Since the attenuation of the sporozoites by X-rays could also be effected by irradiating live infected mosquitoes [20], it became possible to try the method in human volunteers. Three individuals have been vaccinated to *P. falciparum* in this way [21]. Over a period of some weeks each was exposed to the bites of about 1000 irradiated infected mosquitoes and subsequently challenged by the bites of a small number of non-irradiated infected mosquitoes. Each was immune to challenge with either the same or a heterologous strain of *P. falciparum* for a period of about 3 months after the end of the immunization procedure. One of the volunteers, while he was immune to *P. falciparum*, was shown to be fully susceptible to mosquito-transmitted *P. vivax* but was later immunized to this species by exposure to the bites of a large number of infected irradiated mosquitoes. Again the immunity lasted 3–6 months.

A single surface antigen on the sporozoite is the immunogenic agent, as first shown for *P. berghei* through the development of monoclonal antibodies that would confer passive protection in mice against sporozoite challenge [22]. The immunogenic circumsporozoite or CS protein of *P. berghei* has a molecular weight of 44000. Similar CS proteins have now been demonstrated for two species of simian malaria, *P. knowlesi* and *P. cynomolgi*, and for the two human malaria species *P. falciparum* and *P. vivax* [23, 24, 25, 26, 27–30]. Furthermore the genes encoding these last 4 proteins have been cloned and the structures of the polypeptides determined. All have an amino terminal signal-like sequence and a carboxy terminal hydrophobic sequence with several groups of charged residues present in both of these regions. The middle portion of the molecule consists of a series of tandem repeats and it is here that the molecules of the different species differ greatly from each other. As illustrated in Fig. 1, the CS proteins of *P. falciparum* and *P. knowlesi* show marked homology on the regions flanking the repeat sequence but have very different tandem repeats [28]. It is this repeat domain of

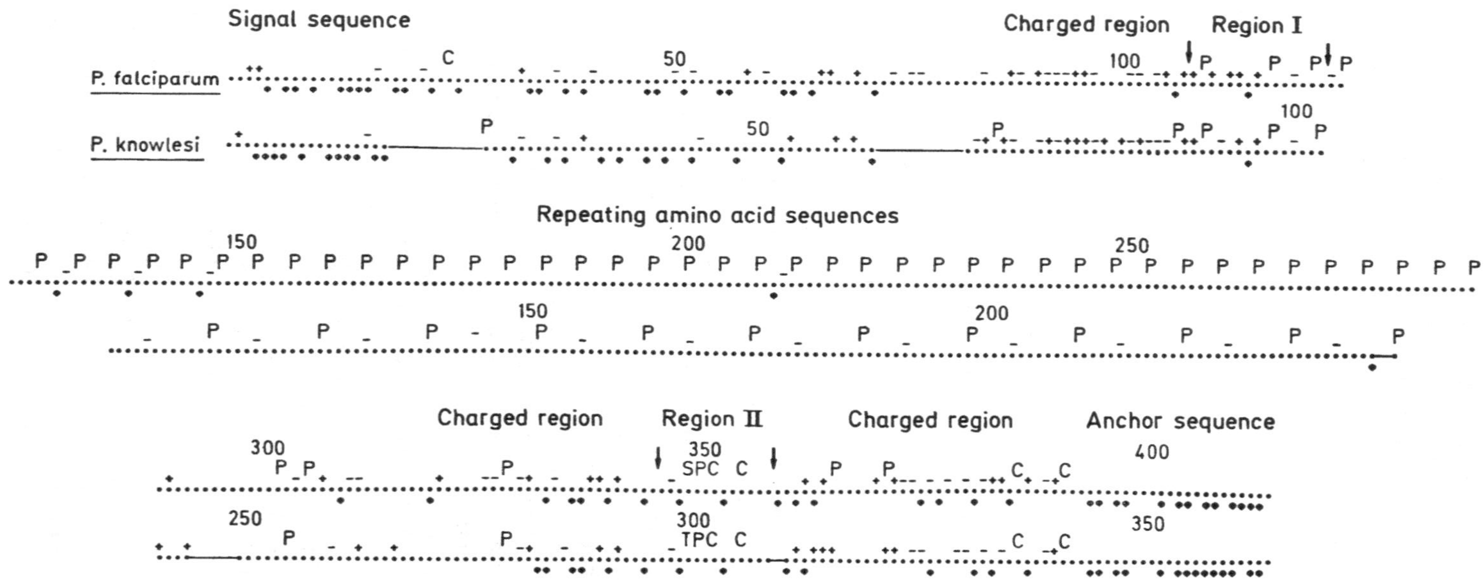

Fig. 1. Circumsporozoite protein structure. The amino acid sequences of the CS proteins of *P. falciparum* and *P. knowlesi* are displayed together in a symbolic form to highlight the various regions of the two proteins and to illustrate their similar structure. The *P. falciparum* sequence is divided into three segments, one preceding and one following the repeating amino acid sequence, and it appears in the figure above the analogous parts of the *P. knowlesi* CS protein sequence. Each amino acid is represented by a filled circle. Since the two proteins differ in length, spaces (indicated with a solid line) were introduced into the *P. knowlesi* sequence in a limited number of places to adjust the alignment. Amino acids carrying a charge at physiological pH are indicated above the line (Asp or Glu as -; Arg or Lys as +). The hydrophobic amino acids Ile, Leu, Phe, Trp, Tyr, or Val are indicated below the line as φ. Pro and Cys are designated with P and C, respectively. The initial three amino acids of the repeating amino acid sequences of *P. knowlesi* are included in the pre-repeat part in this comparison since they form part of region I. Also, the Pro was included after the end of the *P. knowlesi* repeat to illustrate that Pro occurs at this juncture in both proteins. The single amino acid difference in region II is identified as S for Ser in *P. falciparum* and T for Thr in *P. knowlesi*. From Dame et al.[28] with permission from the author and from *Science* (copyright AAAS 1984)

the peptide that is immunodominant accounting for the species specificity of antibody reactivity to the sporozoites. Extensive strain-dependent variation of the repeat sequences has already been found for both simian species *P. knowlesi* and *P. cynomolgi*. Strangely enough this is not the case for *P. vivax* [29], even though its CS gene shows close homology to that of *P. knowlesi*. Fortunately, this also is not the situation with *P. falciparum* (thought to be more closely related on the basis of DNA homology to avian than to simian parasites [31]. All strains of *P. falciparum* so far investigated show the same repeated epitope of 4 amino acids. The complete peptide, as deduced from isolation of the complete CS gene, has 41 tandem repeat tetrapeptides (Fig. 1). Thirty-seven of these are Asn-Ala-Asn-Pro whereas the other four are Asn-Val-Asp-Pro. That the repeat tetrapeptide is the immunodominant epitope has been conclusively demonstrated [32]. Three synthetic peptides were prepared: $(Asn\text{-}Ala\text{-}Asn\text{-}Pro)_2$, which may be abbreviated as $(NANP)_2$, $(NANP)_3$ and $(NANP)_4$. When these were tested for inhibition of binding of monoclonal antibodies to extracts of *P. falciparum* sporozoites, it was found that $(NANP)_2$ was a poor inhibitor whereas $(NANP)_3$ and $(NANP)_4$ both inhibited strongly and to about the same extent. Accordingly the dodecapeptide $(NANP)_3$, was used for further work. Rabbits were immunized with conjugates of $(NANP)_3$ coupled to tetanus toxoid with glutaraldehyde. In animals injected with 1 mg of this antigen together with Freund's incomplete adjuvant antibody titers of 1,000 to 10,000 were attained as measured by a radioactive assay. These antisera reacted with the surface of glutaraldehyde-fixed *P. falciparum* sporozoites in the immunofluorescent reaction and also gave circumsporozoite reactions with the viable sporozoites. One such serum with an IFA titer of 10,000 was shown to neutralize the infectivity of *P. falciparum* sporozoites *in vitro* for the human hepatoma line Hep G2-A16 even at an IgG concentration of only 2 μg/ml [32]. Similar results have been obtained with synthetic peptides conjugated to thyroglobulin [33]. Antibodies to peptides consisting of 8 to 16 residues of the repeat region all produced a circumsporozoite reaction and inhibited invasion of sporozoites *in vitro* whereas antibodies to peptides representing the conserved regions I or II had no biological activity.

Hence the rationale has been established for the *in vivo* testing of such synthetic peptides and of sequences of the CS proteins of *P. falciparum* expressed in *Escherichia coli* [34]. For the latter, the recombinant protein must of course be purified; 60 mg of protein were recovered from 30 g. wet weight of bacteria. Since antibody-eliciting activity of these materials is greatly increased by the use of an adjuvant, it is likely that they will be tested together with aluminum hydroxide, an adjuvant that has been safely used in people. Another possible way of supplying the adjuvant is suggested by results obtained by coupling a conjugate of a synthetic peptide of a portion of the CS protein of *P. knowlesi* and tetanus toxoid with ε-amino caproic murabutide, an analogue of muramyldipeptide [37]. This preparation elicited high titers of anti-peptide antibodies and low titers of anticarrier antibodies. It may also become desirable to express the CS protein in other vehicles. Thus the CS protein of *P. knowlesi* has already been efficiently expressed in the yeast *Saccharomyces cerevisiae* [35]. It has also been expressed by infectious recombinant vaccinia virus [36], but apparently not in such a way as to give good antibody production in vaccinated animals. With further development this might provide a particularly suitable way in which to present a malaria vaccine since methods for handling and storage of vaccinia virus are well known. Meanwhile the trials about to be done in human volunteers should furnish very important information as to antibody levels elicited, whether they are protective, and how long they last. It is important to note that protection against sporozoite challenge by *P. falciparum* would be difficult to test in an animal model. The only susceptible experimental animals, the monkeys *Aotus trivirgatus* and *Saimiri sciureus*, vary greatly in their response to sporozoite inoculation, some being entirely refractory, so that relatively large groups of animals would be needed for a significant result. Even with the best available system of splenectomized *Aotus* from Colombia and the Santa Lucia strain of *P. falciparum* a minimum of 10 animals per test group would be required (W. E. Collins, personal communication).

Since the natural history of malaria in a holoendemic region shows that prolonged repeated reinfection occurs throughout childhood before there is any effective immunity, the sporozoite vaccine, if it is to be effective, will have to give an initial titer of anti-sporozoite antibody sufficient to eliminate most if not all injected sporozoites. Since a single sporozoite can produce some 10,000 preerythrocytic merozoites, against which the sporozoite vaccine gives no protection, it would seem desirable also to induce immunity to the erythrocytic stages.

3 Merozoite Vaccine

It is the erythrocytic stages of the malaria parasite that cause disease. Their development stimulates antibody production; that some of these antibodies are protective has been demonstrated by passive transfer not only in various experimental malarias but also for human falciparum malaria [38]. In addition, however, the numerous antigens of the parasites stimulate the production of antibodies having no relevance to immunity, as well as the formation of an excess of globulins; IgG and IgM levels of West Africans are about 3 times higher than those of Europeans or of Africans long resident in a non-malarious region [39]. This excess is presumed to result not only from direct stimulation of B lymphocytes but also from a malaria-induced defect in suppressive T cells. In an acute attack of *P. falciparum* malaria T cell numbers are decreased and B cells increased and the ratio of T-helper cells to T-suppressive cells is reduced [40]. There may also be other direct immunosuppressive effects [41]. In the complex interplay between the parasites with their many antigenic components and the immunological system of the host, the parasites produce substances that modulate and even suppress immune responses as well as others that stimulate effective immune responses.

The possibility of separating antigens that stimulate an effective immune response from all the others provides the best hope for development of a vaccine against erythrocytic stages. Here most of the work has been done with *P. falciparum*. First it was shown that merozoites obtained either from infected *Aotus* monkeys or from continuous cultures in human erythrocytes would induce immunity in *Aotus* monkeys if administered with an appropriate adjuvant [9,10,11,42]. Note that the New World monkeys *Aotus trivirgatus* and *Saimiri sciureus* can be used for testing erythrocytic stage vaccines since one can prepare in advance by blood passage strains of *P. falciparum* whose erythrocytic stages are adapted to one or the other species of monkey. Three general methods have then been used during the past 10 years to identify specific antigens involved in protective immunity to the erythrocytic stages:

A) Production of monoclonal antibodies and selection for those that inhibit *P. falciparum* growth *in vitro*. The antibody can then be used to localize the corresponding antigen and to isolate it by affinity chromatography.

B) Selection of major antigens, separated by SDS-polyacrylamide gel electrophoresis, that are recognized by hyperimmune serum from either humans or infected monkeys.

C) Identification of functional surface receptors, either those on merozoites involved in erythrocyte invasion or those on schizont-infected erythrocytes involved in sequestration.

Among the numerous antigens so far identified the following appear of special interest. It will be noted that several of these are associated with the merozoite. The tentative localization of those identified so far is shown in Fig. 2.

1. An antigen of about 200,000 relative molecular weight present on the surface membrane of schizonts. This is a predominant antigen recognized by human hyperimmune serum [43]. It is broken down in the formation of merozoites to products of 83000, 42000 and 19000 M_r that are on the surface of the merozoites (Fig. 2). Monoclonal antibodies to the 190–200 kd proteins [44] however inhibit growth *in vitro* only at high concentrations [45]. This is also true for the corresponding antigen of *P. knowlesi* [46]. Partial protection against *P. falciparum* was obtained in *Saimiri* monkeys immunized with the 200 kd protein purified from cultured parasites [47] or prepared after cloning and expression of the corresponding gene in bacteria [48]. This protein shows considerable antigenic diversity among isolates from the same geographic region as well as from different regions. Although each parasite clone produces a

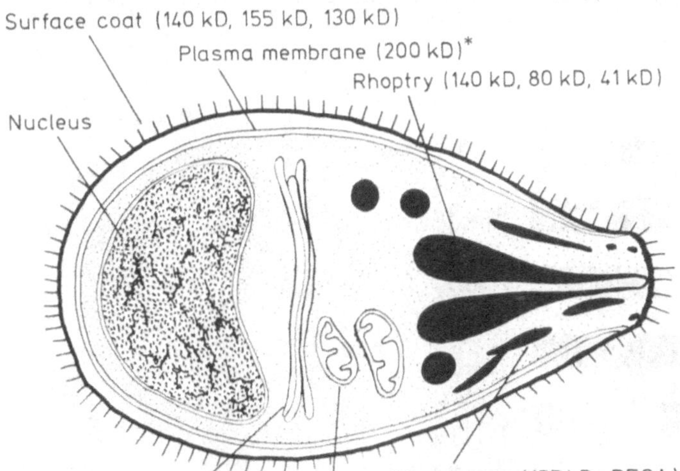

Fig. 2. The localization of merozoite proteins, identified by size (kD), is based on references discussed in text. The major merozoite surface protein (190 kD–200 kD, Ref. [43–50]) appears to be localized on the surface coat but may have an anchor segment in the lipid bilayer and thus may be the protein that attaches the coat to the plasma membrane

protein distinct from the equivalent product in other clones, all of these proteins are immunologically interrelated and have determinants in common. They may eventually provide a useful system for antigenic typing of *P. falciparum* [49]. The primary structure of this protein has been deduced from the nucleotide sequence of cDNA and genomic clones covering the complete coding sequence [50]. It does not show an extensive repeat domain but has a consensus anchor sequence at the C-terminal end. This suggests the C-terminal end is inserted in or through the plasma membrane of the merozoite, whereas the N-terminal extends into the coat.

2. A protein of M_r 140,000, also from late schizonts and merozoites. This was identified by a monoclonal antibody that inhibited growth *in vitro* [52,53]. In a comparative experiment it gave a somewhat better immunization of *Saimiri* monkeys than did the 195 kd protein [47]. It is a major soluble secreted antigen [54].

3. A protein of M_r 41,000 also identified by a monoclonal antibody that inhibited growth *in vitro* [51,52,53]. When this protein was purified by affinity chromatography and used to vaccinate 4 *Saimiri* monkeys (together with Freund's adjuvant) the challenge infections showed peak parasitemias of only 1%, 0.2%, 0.08% and 0.05% reached on days 12, 34, 35 and 28 respectively, whereas the 4 controls had peaks of 11%, 12%, > 20% and > 20% reached on days 10, 20, 10 and 16 respectively (Perrin — personal communication). This protein is apparently derived from the apical organelles of merozoites which almost surely play an essential role in the invasion process (Fig. 2). It deserves and is receiving much further attention.

4. Two proteins that bind to erythrocyte glycophorin and are on the surface of the merozoite (Fig. 2). Since it has been shown that the erythrocyte receptor for merozoites is glycophorin A plus B [55,56], these two proteins are the presumed corresponding receptors on the merozoites responsible for attachment to human erythrocytes. The proteins are of M_r 155,000 and 130,000 [57]. Antibodies to them block invasion

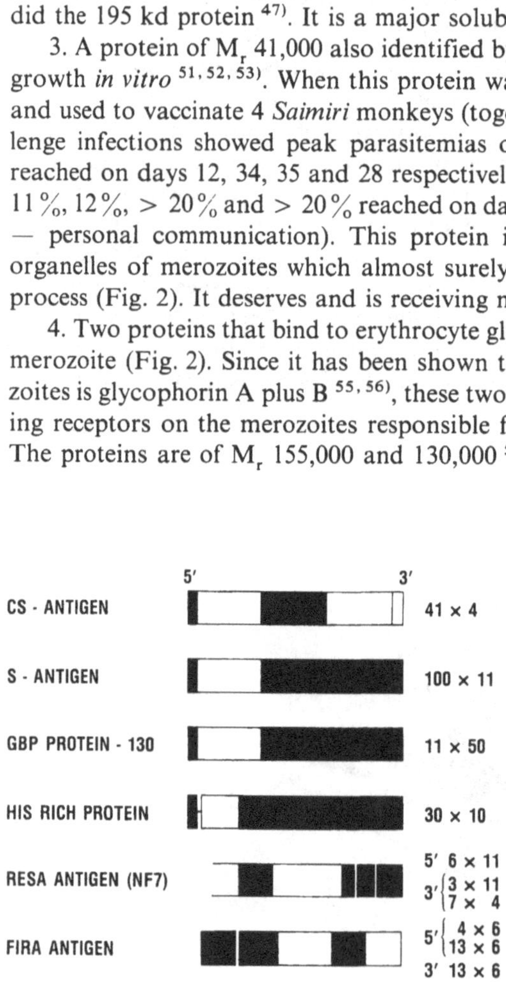

Fig. 3. Gene organization of *P. falciparum* and *P. lophurae* antigens. CS antigen [28]; S-antigen [76]; GBP protein [59]; his rich protein, *P. lophurae* [74]; RESA antigen [64]; FIRA antigen [65]. The dark areas denote the region of repeat domains and the number of repeats and amino acids is given for each block, starting from the 3′ end. The structure of RESA antigen and FIRA is not complete

in vitro. The gene for the 130 kd glycophorin binding protein has been isolated and sequenced [58]. It contains 11 tandem repeats of a 50 amino acid sequence which binds to glycophorin (Fig. 3) [59]. Monoclonal antibody against the repeats expressed in *E. coli* significantly blocked merozoite invasion [60]. There are as yet no reports of attempts to immunize with these interesting materials. The gene for the 130 kd glycophorin-binding protein is conserved in 4 geographically diverse isolates (Perkins — personal communication) as is the epitope recognized by polyclonal antibodies raised against the *E. coli*-expressed fusion protein.

5. A protein of M_r 155,000 that has been localized to the micronemes and rhoptries of merozoites [61] rather than their surface. This protein which is identified in merozoites by immunoflorescence using hyperimmune serum, cannot be found on the newly formed ring soon after invasion of an erythrocyte; instead it appears on the surface of the newly invaded erythrocyte [62, 61]. It has therefore been named the ring-infected erythrocyte surface antigen (RESA). Monoclonal antibody to it, as well as affinity purified human immunglobulin from malarial serum, blocks growth of the parasite *in vitro* [63]. Again, no tests of immunization have yet been reported. Because of its presence in micronemes and rhoptries, this protein may be involved in invasion processes that follow attachment. Once the ring stage has formed the protein can be shown by immunoelectron microscopy only on the surface of the erythrocyte. How it gets there and what it does there are problems for the future. The gene for the RESA protein has been cloned and sequenced; once again there is a complex tandem repeat structure [64] (Fig. 3).

6. A protein somewhat resembling RESA but having an M_r of about 300,000 and occurring probably in the parasitophorous vacuole as well as in merozoites [65]. This is apprently a dominant immunogen since a cDNA clone, Ag 231, expressing the antigen in *E. coli* reacted with about 90% of sera from a group of 65 people from New Guinea, an endemic region for *P. falciparum*. The structure of the protein as predicted from the nucleotide sequence is most interesting (Fig. 3). At the 5′ end it has 4 repeats of 6 amino acids each (Block I) followed by Block II consisting of 13 inexact repeats of another 6 amino acids. There follows a highly charged region of 81 amino acids followed in turn by Block III consisting of 13 inexact repeats of 6 amino acids very similar to those of Block II but more variable. Finally there is another charged region quite similar to the first. This protein has been termed FIRA for falciparum interspersed repeat antigen.

7. Parasite proteins concerned in sequestration. During almost the entire latter half of the 48 hr growth cycle *P. falciparum* parasites are not found in the circulating blood; instead they are sequestered in capillaries of organs where they adhere to the endothelial cells. In this way they are protected from having to go through the spleen where they could be recognized and destroyed. The adherence to endothelial cells is mediated by special protuberances or knobs on the surface of the infected erythrocytes that appear as the parasite becomes a trophozoite and become more numerous as it matures. These knobs are essential to adherence [66] but not sufficient [67]. Antisera block adherence *in vitro* and sequestration *in vivo* [68,69,70]. A knob protein of 90,000 M_r has been identified in a number of strains [71, 67] but there is no evidence that antibody to this blocks sequestration. The knob protein does not appear to be exposed on the erythrocyte surface. Since this is a histidine-rich protein it is relevant here to mention the first pure protein obtained from any malaria parasite, the histidine-rich protein

from the avian malaria *P. lophurae* [72, 73, 74]. The gene for this protein has been cloned; it again shows repeating units [74].

8. The S-antigens, heat stable proteins (to 5 min at 100 °C), were first demonstrated in the serum of malarious patients [75]. They show great antigenic diversity; each isolate of *P. falciparum* has a characteristic S-antigen, but they do contain a region of sequence homology [76]. They range in molecular weight from 130 to 250 kd, largely as a result of the different number of tandem repeats. These antigens are found in the culture fluid of *in vitro* cultures as well as patients' plasma and are derived from the parasitophorous vacuole. The gene has been localized to chromosome 7 in pulsed field gradient electrophoresis, whereas the RESA gene is on chromosome 1 [15].

On the basis of present limited information, the antigens described in Sections 3, 4 and 5 above seem most promising, either because they have been shown to give excellent protection against heterologous challenge (Sect. 3) or because they do not vary from one isolate to another. This picture may change as additional antigens are tested for protective immunity to challenge by live erythrocytic parasites in *Aotus* or *Saimiri* monkeys.

Cell-mediated immunity. The foregoing discussion has been concerned with antigens that stimulate the formation of protective antibody. This does not imply that cell-mediated immunity plays a minor role. Indeed it has been shown that the development of antisporozoite antibodies, at least in mice, is thymus dependent [77]. Furthermore, in rodent malaria T cell-dependent immunity against the erythrocytic stages is more important than antibody-dependent immunity. Thus T cell-deprived or nude mice cannot control and recover from infection with *P. yoelii*, a species of malaria not lethal to normal mice. Again with *P. yoelii* it has been found that an immunogenic blood stage antigen of 230,000 molecular weight greatly stimulated both helper T cells and T cells responsible for delayed hypersensitivity in mice vaciinated with it [78]. That T cells are important also in primate malaria is indicated by the need for Freund's complete adjuvant, or certain substitutes for it, in order to get successful vaccination against erythrocytic stages with killed merozoites of *P. knowlesi* in rhesus monkeys or *P. falciparum* in *Aotus* monkeys [4].

T cells probably act in a number of ways. They may stimulate macrophages to ingest infected erythrocytes. They could increase the activity of natural killer (NK) cells. The NK cells in turn could exert antiparasitic effects via lymphokines. Macrophages also secrete a number of products directly toxic to the parsites, including oxidative enzymes such as glucose oxidase and polyamine oxidase. Human monocytes activated by γ-interferon exerted a killing effect on *P. falciparum* in culture, which was largely but not entirely, associated with the release of H_2O_2 [79, 80]. Serum from animals containing tumor necrosis factor is toxic to malaria parasites *in vitro* [81] but the purified TNF has no action. Furthermore, immune sera from the Sudan that inhibited intra-erythrocytic growth of *P. falciparum* lacked TNF activity [82]. A study of the effects on *P. falciparum in vitro* of mononuclear cells and serum from Gambian children in different stages of infection with *P. falciparum* has revealed some interesting results [83]. Sera from acutely infected children were not inhibitory whereas those from children recovering from an attack were, some from convalescent children inhibiting growth by 50%. This humoral response was more effective against the most recent infecting parasite strain than against other isolates. On the other hand, mononuclear cell cytotoxicity was equally effective against all strains. Although mononuclear cells plus serum from acutely ill children had some inhibitory effect, the parsite-killing was most effective with cells and serum from children with low grade infections of at least 10 days duration. Mononuclear cells from uninfected children together with autologous serum, taken during the season of minimal malaria transmission, had no effect. The monocytemediated effect kills the parasites within the red cells and presumably results from soluble products released by adherent cells (Brown, Greenwood & Terry, unpublished). Studies of this type will be of special importance in following the effects of early trials of merozoite vaccines.

In view of all the indications for the role of cell-mediated immunity it is likely that all vaccines to be tested will be administered with an adjuvant. Aluminum hydroxide is the only adjuvant universally accepted as safe for human use, but many others are under development [84, 85].

Antigamete or Transmission-blocking Vaccine. This would be of no direct benefit to the person receiving it, since it would not block the sporozoite or erythrocytic stages. It would however help to interrupt transmission in the mosquito, so that its action would be like that of the gametocytocidal drug primaquine. Such interruption of transmission can be a major factor in an integrated malaria control program, especially where it is essential to try to stop further transmission of drug-resistant falciparum malaria. A transmission-blocking vaccine would be administered together with a sporozoite vaccine or a merozoite vaccine or with both.

Antibodies induced in the vertebrate host to gametes or zygotes, which normally never occur in the vertebrate host, will act in the midgut of a mosquito that feeds on such a host to inactivate gametes or zygotes resulting from gametocytes taken up with the same blood meal. This kind of action, first shown and studied in some detail with the avian parasite *P. gallinaceum* [86] has since been demonstrated in *P. falciparum* [16, 87], using gametocytes from cultures infective to mosquitoes. Several antigens have been identified by reactivity with monoclonal antibodies that block mosquito infection, reducing the average number of oocysts by 95 to 100% [88]. Of special interest are antigens of the 48/45 kd doublet and of 25 kd. The former are present in gametocytes and are later expressed on the surface of newly formed macrogametes. Monoclonal antibodies to this doublet block formation of ookinetes; presumably they interfere with fertilization of the macrogametes. These proteins are no longer present on the surface of ookinetes. The 25 kd protein is also already present in mature gametocytes. It is however barely detectable on the surface of newly emerged macrogametes, becoming progessively expressed during the next two hours. A monoclonal antibody to this protein did not prevent ookinete formation, yet it gave a 95% reduction in oocyst yield. Perhaps the 25 kd protein has a role in penetration of the mosquito midgut by the ookinete.

It is remarkable that antibodies to these proteins have been found naturally ocurring in the sera of a few individuals long resident in holoendemic malarious regions. Presumably this results from prolonged exposure to gametocytes. One such serum was shown to block transmission, supporting the feasibility of induction of such an immunity (Meeuwissen — personal communication).

4 Conclusion

For the moment, one can only agree with B. M. Greenwood's "View from the bush" [89] that "recent developments in our understanding of the molecular biology and immunology of the malaria parasite have so far contributed little to the practical problems of malaria in Africa." At the same time, however, it is clear that the possibilities for development of effective vaccines are so great as to warrant a certain optimism. As Greenwood again has emphasized, it will be important to encourage early field trials rather than delay in the hope of getting some more nearly perfect preparation. Every year perhaps a million children die of falciparum malaria. Every year drug resistance spreads to new regions. The situation is urgent and the performance of field trals difficult and time-consuming. In the next few years we can look forward at the least to important and valuable results, and perhaps to exciting ones.

5 References

1. McGregor, I. A.: Trans. Roy. Soc. Trop. Med. Hyg. *58*, 80 (1964)
2. Peters, W.: Antimalarial Drugs, p. 423, Berlin-Heidelberg-New York, Springer 1984
3. Cohen, S.: Proc. Roy. Soc. Lond. B *202*, 323 (1979)
4. Cohen, S.: Br. Med. Bull. *38* (2), 161 (1982)
5. Cohen, S., Butcher, G. A. & Crandell, R. B.: Nature *223*, 368 (1969)
6. Phillips, R. S., Trigg, R. J., Scott-Finnigan, T. J. & Bartholomew, R. K.: Parasitology *65*, 525 (1972)
7. Reese, R. T. & Motyl, M. R.: J. Immunol. *123*, 1894 (1979)
8. Brown, G. V., Anders, R. F. & Knowles, G.: Infec. Immun. *39*, 1228 (1983)
9. Mitchell, G. H., Richards, W. H. G., Butcher, G. A. & Cohen, S.: Lancet *1*, 1335 (1977)
10. Siddiqui, W. A.: Science *197*, 388 (1977)
11. Reese, R. T., Trager, W., Jensen, J. B., Miller, D. A. & Tantravahi, P.: Proc. Natl. Acad. Sci. USA *75*, 5665 (1978)
12. Trager, W. & Jensen, J. B.: Science *193*, 673 (1976)
13. Trager, W. & Jensen, J. B.:Nature *273*, 621 (1978)
14. Trager, W., Tershakovec, M., Lyandvert, L., Stanley, H., Lanners, N. & Gubert, E.: Proc. Natl. Acad. Sci. USA *78*, 10 (1981)
15. Kemp, D. J., Corcoran, L. M., Coppel, R. L., Stahl, H. D., Bianco, A. E., Brown, G. V., & Anders, R. F.: Nature *315*, 347 (1985)
16. Vermeulen, A. N., Ponnedurai, T., Beckers, P. J. A., Verhave, J.-P., Smiths, M. A. & Meuwissen, J. E. H. Th.: J. Exp. Med. *162*, 1460 (1985)
17. Milstein, C.: Eur. J. Biochem. *118*, 429 (1981)
18. Russell, P. & Mohan, B. N.: J. Exper. Med. *76*, 477 (1942)
19. Nussenzweig, R. S., Vanderberg, J. & Most, H.: Mil. Med. (suppl.) *134*, 1176 (1969)
20. Vanderberg, J. P., Nussenzweig, R. S. & Most, H.: J. Parasitol. *56*, 350 (1970)
21. Clyde, D. F., McCarthy, V. C., Miller, R. M. & Woodward, W. E.: Am. J. Trop. Med. Hyg. *24*, 397 (1975)
22. Potocnjak, P., Yoshida, N., Nussenzweig, R. S. & Nussenzweig, V.: J. Exp. Med. *151*, 1504 (1980)
23. Ellis, J., Ozaki, L. S., Gwadz, R. W., Cochrane, A. H., Nussenzweig, V., Nussenzweig, R. S. & Godson, G. N.: Nature *302*, 536 (1983)
24. Ozaki, L. S., Svec, P., Nussenzweig, R. S., Nussenzweig, V. & Godson, G. N.: Cell *34*, 815 (1983)
25. Sharma, S., Svec, P., Mitchell, G. H. & Godson, G. N.: Science *229*, 779 (1985)
26. Enea, V., Arnot, D., Schmidt, E. C., Cochrane, A., Gwadz, R. & Nussenzweig, R. S.: Proc. Natl. Acad. Sci. USA *81*, 7520 (1984)

27. Enea, V., Ellis, J., Zavala, F., Arnot, D. E., Asavanich, A., Quakyi, I. & Nussenzweig, R. S.: Science *225*, 628 (1984)
28. Dame, J. B., Williams, J. L., McCutchan, T. F., Weber, J. L., Wirtz, R. A., Hockmeyer, W. T., Maloy, W. L., Haynes, J. D., Schneider, I., Roberts, D., Sanders, G. S., Reddy, E. P., Diggs, C. L. & Miller, L. H.: Science *225*, 593 (1984)
29. Arnot, D. E., Barnwell, J. W., Tam, J. P., Nussenzweig, V., Nussenzweig, R. S. & Enea, V.: Science *230*, 815 (1985)
30. McCutchan, T. F., Lal, A. A., de la Cruz, V. F., Miller, L. H., Maloy, W. L., Charoenvit, Y., Beaudoin, R. L., Guerry, P., Wistar, R., Jr., Hoffman, S. L., Hockmeyer, W. T., Collins, W. E. & Wirth, D.: Science *230*, 1381 (1985)
31. McCutchan, T. F., Dame, J. B., Miller, L. H. & Barnwell, J. W.: Science *225*, 808 (1984)
32. Zavala, F., Tam, J. P., Hollingdale, M. A., Cochrane, A. H., Quakyi, I., Nussenzweig, R. S. & Nussenzweig, V.: Science *228*, 1436 (1985)
33. Ballou, W. R., Rothbard, J., Wirtz, R. A., Gordon, D. M., Williams, J. S., Gore, R. W., Schneider, I., Hollingdale, M. R., Beaudoin, R. L., Maloy, W. L., Miller, L. H. & Hockmeyer, W. T.: Science *228*, 996 (1985)
34. Young, J. F., Hockmeyer, W. T., Gross, M., Ballou, W. R., Wirtz, R. A., Trosper, J. H., Beaudoin, R. L., Hollingdale, M. R., Miller, L. H., Diggs, C. L. & Rosenberg, M.: Science *228*, 958 (1985)
35. Sharma, S. & Godson, G. N.: Science *228*, 879 (1985)
36. Smith, G. L., Godson, G. N., Nussenzweig, V., Nussenzweig, R. S., Barnwell, J. & Moss, B.: Science *224*, 397 (1984)
37. Clough, E. R., Jolivet, M., Audibert, P., Barnwell, J. W., Schlesinger, D. H. & Chedid, L.: Biochem. Biophys. Res. Comm. *131*, 70 (1985)
38. Cohen, S., McGregor, I. A. & Carrington, S.: Nature *192*, 733 (1961)
39. Cohen, S. & Lambert, P. H.: Immunology of Parasitic Infections, p. 422, Oxford, Blackwell Scientific 1982²
40. Whittle, H. C., Brown, J., March, K., Greenwood, B. M., Seidelin, P., Tighe, H. & Wedderburn, L.: Nature *312*, 449 (1984)
41. Williamson, W. A. & Greenwood, B. M.: Lancet *1(8078)*, 1328 (1978)
42. Trager, W., Lanners, H. N., Stanley, H. A. & Langreth, S. G.: Parasite Immunol. *5*, 225 (1983)
43. Holder, A. A. & Freeman, R. R.: J. Exp. Med. *156*, 1528 (1982)
44. Hall, R. J., McBride, J., Morgan, G., Tait, A., Zolg, J. W. & Walliker, D.: Mol. Bioechem. Parasitol. *7*, 247 (1983)
45. Pirson, P. J. & Perkins, M. E.: J. Immunol. *134*, 1946 (1985)
46. Epstein, N., Miller, L. H., Kaushel, D. C., Udeinya, I. J., Rener, J., Howard, R. J., Asofsky, R., Aikawa, M. & Hess, R. L.: J. Immunol. *127*, 212 (1981)
47. Perrin, L. H., Merkl, B., Loche, M., Chizzolini, C., Smart, J. & Richle, R.: J. Exp. Med. *160*, 441 (1984)
48. Hall, R., Hyde, J. E., Goman, M., Simmons, D. L., Hope, I. A., Mackey, M., Scaife, J., Merkli, B., Richle, R. & Stocker, J.: Nature *311*, 379 (1984)
49. McBride, J. S., Newbold, C. I. & Anand, R.: J. Exp. Med. *161*, 160 (1985)
50. Holder, A. A., Lockyer, M. J., Odink, K. G., Sandhu, J. S., Riveros-Moreno, V., Nicholls, S. C., Hillman, Y., Darey, L. S., Tizard, M. L. V., Schwarz, R. T. & Freeman, R. R.: Nature *317*, 270 (1985)
51. Perrin, L. H., Ramirez, E., Liu E-H & Lambert, P. H.: Clin. Exp. Immun. *41*, 91 (1980)
52. Perrin, L. H., Ramirez, E., Lambert, P. H. & Miescher, P. A.: Nature *289*, 291 (1981)
53. Perrin, L. H. & Dayal, R.: Immunol. Rev. *61*, 245 (1982)
54. Perrin, L. H., Loche, M., Dedet, J-P, Rousilhon, C. & Fandeur, T.: Clin. Exp. Immunol. *56*, 67 (1984)
55. Perkins, M.: J. Cell Biol. *90*, 563 (1981)
56. Pasvol, G. J. S., Wainscoat, J. S. & Weatherall, D. J.: Nature *297*, 64 (1982)
57. Perkins, M. E.: J. Exp. Med. *160*, 788 (1984)
58. Ravetch, J. V., Kochan, J. & Perkins, M. E.: Science *227*, 1593 (1985)
59. Kochan, J., Perkins, M. & Ravetch, J. (in press)
60. Perkins, M. & Ravetch, R.: Modern Approaches to Vaccines, CSH Press (in press) (1986)

61. Brown, G. V., Culvenor, J. G., Crewther, P. E., Bianco, A. E., Coppel, R. L., Saint, R. B., Stahl, H-D, Kemp, D. J. & Anders, R. F.: J. Exp. Med. *162*, 774 (1985)
62. Masuda, A. et al. (in press)
63. Perlmann, H., Berzins, K., Wahlgren, M., Carlsson, J., Bjorkmann, A., Patarroyo, M. E. & Perlmann, P.: J. Exp. Med. *159*, 1686 (1984)
64. Coppel, R. L., Cowman, A. F., Anders, R. F., Bianco, A. E., Saint, R. B., Lingelbach, K. R., Kemp, D. J. & Brown, G. V.: Nature *310*, 789 (1984)
65. Stahl, H.-D., Crewther, P. E., Anders, R. F., Brown, G. V., Coppel, R. L., Bianco, A. E., Mitchell, G. F. & Kemp, D. J.: Proc. Natl. Acad. Sci. USA *82*, 543 (1984)
66. Raventos-Suarez, C., Kaul, D. K., Macaluso, F. & Nagel, R. L.: Proc. Natl. Acad. Sci. USA *82*, 3829 (1985)
67. Leech, J. H., Barnwell, J. W., Aikawa, M., Miller, L. H. & Howard, R. J.: J. Cell Biol. *98*, 1256 (1984)
68. Udeinya, I. J., Miller, L. H., McGregor, I. A. & Jensen, J. B.: Nature *303*, 429 (1983)
69. David, P. H., Hommel, M., Miller, L. H., Udeinya, I. J. & Oligino, L. D.: Proc. Natl. Acad. Sci. USA *80*, 5075 (1983)
70. Hommel, M., David, P. H. & Oligino, L. D.: J. Exp. Med. *157*, 1137 (1983)
71. Kilejian, A.: Proc. Natl. Acad. Sci. USA *76*, 4650 (1979)
72. Kilejian, A.: J. Biol. Chem. *249*, 4650 (1974)
73. Kilejian, A., Chen, S. & Sloma, A.: Mol. Biochem. Parasitol. *14*, 1 (1985)
74. Ravetch, J. V., Feder, R., Pavlovec, A. & Blobel, G.: Nature *312*, 616 (1984)
75. Wilson, R. J. M., McGregor, I. A. & Williams, K.: Trans. Roy. Soc. Trop. Med. Hyg. *69*, 453 (1975)
76. Cowman, A. F., Saint, R. B., Coppel, R. L., Brown, G. V., Anders, R. F. & Kemp, D. J.: Cell *40*, 775 (1985)
77. Nussenzweig, R. S., Cochrane, A. H. & Lustig, H. J.: Rodent Malaria, p. 248, New York, Academic Press 1978
78. Playfair, J. H. L., de Souza, J. B., Freeman, R. R. & Holder, A. A.: Clin. Exp. Immunol. *62*, 19 (1985)
79. Ockenhouse, C. F., Schulman, S. & Shear, H. L.: J. Immunol. *133*, 1601 (1984)
80. Kharazmi, A., Jepsen, S. & Valerius, N. H.: Scan. J. Immunol. *20*, 93 (1984)
81. Taverne, J., Matthews, N., Depledge, P. & Playfair, J. H. L.: Clin. Exp. Immunol. *57*, 293 (1984)
82. Vande Waa, J. A., Jensen, J. B., Akood, M. A. S. & Bayoumi, R.: Infec. Immun. *45*, 505 (1984)
83. Brown, J. & Greenwood, B. M.: Parasite Immunol. *7*, 265 (1985)
84. Leclerc, C., Morin, A. & Chedid, L.: Rec. Adv. Clin. Immunol. *3*, 187 (1983)
85. Fudenberg, H. H. & Whitten, H. D.: Ann. Rev. Pharmacol. & Toxicol. *24* (1984)
86. Kaushal, D. C., Carter, R., Rener, J., Grotendorst, C. A., Miller, L. H. & Howard, R. J.: J. Immunol. *131*, 2557 (1983)
87. Carter, R., Bushell, G., Saul, A., Graves, P. M. & Kidson, C.: Infec. Immun. *50*, 102 (1985)
88. Greenwood, B. M.: Parasite Immunol *7*, 191 (1985)

Controlled Drug Delivery

Abraham Rubinstein[1] **and Joseph R. Robinson**

School of Pharmacy, University of Wisconsin, Madison, Wisconsin 73706, U.S.A.

The article provides an overview of the present status of controlled drug delivery with an emphasis on some of the future trends that are likely to emerge in this area. To date the primary focus of the field has been the dosage form and drug, which do have a significant bearing on performance of these systems but must be considered in light of the biological barriers that are present. These barriers can include physiological and anatomical aspects of the route of administration as well as the patient status and pathology of the disease to be treated. It is clear that an important element of properly optimizing drug delivery systems is a thorough understanding of these biological barriers and this is a primary focus of investigators in this field.

[1] Visiting Professor, Hebrew University, Jerusalem, Israel

1 Introduction

1.1 Historical Development

Since the late 1960's and early 1970's the area of drug delivery has been involved in a noisy revolution with considerable publicity regarding the therapeutic and economic potential of controlled drug delivery systems. Several events have led to this renewed interest in drug delivery:

- a growing realization in tumor treatment of the significant need to localize cytostatic/cytocidal drugs in specific organs or subset of cells within these organs, i.e., to be able to spatially locate drugs;
- increasing evidence that minimization of tissue drug fluctuations can minimize/eliminate both short and long term side effects to certain drugs;
- the considerable expense and time to bring a new molecule from discovery to the market, estimated to be on the average of 100 million dollars and 12 years, and concomitant shift of some resources to drug delivery.

Despite the interest and the investment in this area of controlled drug delivery the actual marketed success of significantly improved therapeutic delivery systems todate remains relatively small. As a result, the noise of the revolution has decreased but the effort to optimize drug therapy through improved drug delivery remains, given that the potential is still substantial.

The idea of controlling the input of drug to the body was put on a quantitative basis by Teorell in 1937 [1] when he differentiated between "controllable" input concepts and "uncontrollable" elimination processes. Despite this early quantitative model for release of drug from a dosage form, application of these principles took almost two decades.

Attempts to delay the release of drugs to the gastrointestinal tract were described in the literature as early as 1884 [2], when Unna discussed enteric coating of pills using keratin. Indeed, up to the early 1950's, most delayed release dosage forms were based on enteric coating or heavy sugar coating and the intent was to delay release of drug until the dosage form had cleared the stomach and entered the small intestine. Some of these early techniques used coatings that contained an initial priming dose in the coat, intended to be released in the stomach, with the remainder intended for release into the intestine. In practise, such systems were significantly influenced by the physiology and local mileau of the gastrointestinal tract so that in some cases both fractions released drug simultaneously [3]. The first commercially successful sustained release product was the Spansule® capsule by Smith Kline and French Laboratories, introduced in the early 1950's. It contained four fractions of coated particles, each fraction designed to release its contents at two hour intervals so that an approximate continuous release of drug occurred.

Through the remainder of the 1950's and 1960's a variety of sustained release drug delivery systems were introduced to the market. These systems employed coated particles, drug imbedded in a matrix, ion-exchange resins, swelling hydrogels and other relatively primitive technical approaches. The primary thrust of these systems was to extend drug levels in biological fluids and tissues, primarily the blood, without significant concern over constancy of the drug levels over a time course. The term *controlled release* came into vogue in the early 1970's when it became technically possible to exert better control over drug release from a delivery system so that relatively constant drug blood levels resulted. Given the absence of a standard as to what constitutes an invariant drug blood level, the term controlled release and its companion controlled drug delivery system has been badly abused over the past decade and virtually all prolonged release systems now call themselves controlled drug delivery systems.

The companion aspect of control of the rate of drug delivery is control over location of the the drug, i.e., spatial placement in the body. Numerous approaches have been reported in the literature as possible means to improve localization of drugs in certain organs or tissues of the body, i.e., targetting. These approaches include liposomes, loaded red blood cells, nanoparticles, recognition factors attached to the surface of delivery systems, e.g., monoclonal antibodies, low density lipoproteins, sugars, etc.

It is not particularly difficult to deliver drugs specifically to the reticuloendothelial system, the so-called housekeeping organs of the body, the liver, spleen, lungs and bone marrow, since these organs will normally sequester foreign particles from the blood stream. However, achieving specificity for one or more of these organs, or other organs of the body, while at the same time exerting some degree of control over the kinetics of drug release, is considerably more difficult.

1.2 Definitions

When attempting to define controlled release dosage forms, one encounters an enormous variation in descriptive terms, many of which give absolutely no hint as to the nature of the drug delivery system. Thus, terms such as prolonged release, extended release, delayed action, long action, depot, timed release, smart systems, etc., are representative and commonly used terms. Since the distinction between these dosage forms resides with the specific delivery system used rather than individual drugs, a consistent terminology has been suggested [4)]:

Modified release dosage forms — Using conventional or immediate release dosage forms as a reference, all other dosage forms are modified release systems.

a. *Delayed release* — dosage forms that significantly delay drug release after it has been administered to the body, e.g., enteric coated tablets.
b. *Sustained release* — dosage forms that prolong drug levels in biological fluids. Constant drug blood levels are not observed.
c. *Controlled release* — dosage forms that release drug at a constant, or predictable, rate. The blood drug level should be invariant with time.
d. *Organ targetted release* — Dosage forms that release drug to a target organ, The Ocusert® system to deliver pilocarpine to treat glaucoma is an example of an organ targetted system.
e. *Cell or receptor specific release* — Dosage forms that deliver drug at the cellular level, preferably to a specific receptor.

Note that there is no designation for drug delivery systems that target drugs to a specific location and simultaneously provide for control over the rate of drug release

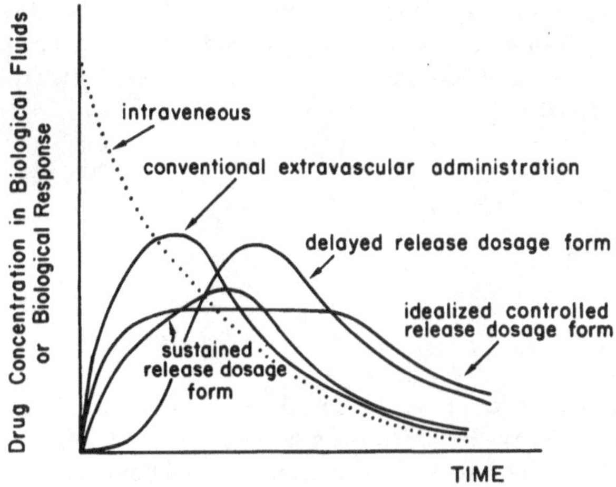

Fig. 1. Theoretical drug profiles in biological fluids assuming first order linear pharmacokinetics, and assuming a linear correlation between drug concentration and biological response, after extravascular administration of four types of drug delivery systems. IV administration is shown for comparison

from the system. There are at present no such drug delivery systems but presumably combinations of the above designations would suffice to describe such systems.

Figure 1 illustrates theoretical drug levels in biological fluids or tissues for four types of drug delivery systems as defined above. A curve for intraveneous drug administration is shown for reference purposes.

1.3 Optimization of Drug Utilization

One of the goals of controlled drug delivery is to achieve optimization of drug use. In general, optimization implies what is desirable and what is achievable within the limits of technical capabilities and inherent physiological constraints.

Optimization with respect to drug delivery implies:

— delivery of intact drug to its target site as quickly as possible;
— maintaining therapeutic drug levels at the target site for as long as desired.
— having drug at the biophase only when it is needed.

There are no drug delivery systems that presently fulfill the above objectives and perhaps the closest is the "artificial pancreas" where the availability of insulin to treat diabetis is controlled by an implantable pump with feedback control that responds to circulating glucose [5,6]. The lack of suitable examples in this regard signals the inherent complexity associated with the problem. Thus, in controlled drug delivery there are considerable constraints imposed by the physico-chemical-biological properties of the drug, the route of drug administration, disease state and general state of the patient, or lack of sophistication regarding the drug delivery system.

The dual difficulty of having control over the rate of drug release from a delivery system while simultaneously trying to target to a specific organ or cell has been prohibitive. Typically, therefore, most commercial sustained/controlled dosage forms do not exhibit serious attempts to truly optimize in this regard, and less then optimum delivery systems are commonly produced and introduced to the market.

Since design of optimized drug delivery systems is complex, a substantial number of experiments are needed to fully explore and assess the many variables influencing its performance. To reduce the number of experiments, a number of mathematical methods have recently been described [7,8].

2 Theory of Controlled Drug Delivery

2.1 Rate Considerations

Most pharmaceutical dosage forms are designed to be administered into a body orifice, and to release drug to that cavity. Released drug is then absorbed into the general circulation for transport to a distant receptor site. Conventional dosage forms release their drug rather promptly and are designed so that the rate limiting step is drug absorption across the biological tissue. In controlled release systems, drug is released slowly into the body and thus the rate limiting step shifts from absorption to release of drug from the drug delivery system.

In essence, the rate of drug release from the delivery system determines the rate of drug availability to the general circulation as well as persistance of drug in the biological fluid.

Elementary model. The persistence of drug in the body, and consequently the duration of drug effect, depends on the drug elimination kinetics, which in turn is governed by body clearance, and the volume space in which the drug is located, the so-called apparent volume of distribution. The pharmacokinetic parameters that characterize the drug's persistence are the elimination rate constant (k elimination) or its inverse value: the mean residence time (MRT). When administered intravenously, a drug's MRT is commonly expressed as follows:

$$MRT_{i.v.} = 1/k_e \tag{1}$$

where k_e is the overall elimination rate constant, assuming first-order kinetics [9].

To relate the MRT to a controlled release model, an absorption phase must be included. An absorption phase is present whenever an extravascular route of administration is used, e.g., the oral route. This absorption is also typical to the kinetics involved when a controlled release dosage form is evaluated. Assuming first-order absorption, the concentration of drug in the blood (C_b) after oral administration is usually described by a biexponential equation. While the first exponent describes the elimination phase, the other is related to the absorption phase as follows:

$$C_b = KF(e^{-k_e t} - e^{-k_a t}) \tag{2}$$

where F is the fraction of dose absorbed, k_e is the overall elimination rate constant, k_a is the absorption rate constant, and K is a proportionality constant.

The relationship between the Mean Residence Time of drug following oral administration and the absorption rate constant is:

$$MRT_{oral} = MRT_{i.v.} + 1/k_a \tag{3}$$

Although MRT_{oral} is expected to be greater than $MRT_{i.v.}$ due to the absorption process, for most conventional drug delivery systems, they are approximately the same, and thus the duration of effect is mostly influenced by the drug's elimination kinetics. For sustained release dosage forms, increasing the value of k_a, by decreasing the release rate of drug from the dosage form, simultaneously results in an increase of MRT_{oral}.

Assuming that the time course of drug in the body parallels its biological response, the simplest way to achieve control over body drug levels is to put drug back into the body at the same rate it is being eliminated e.g., intraveneous drip. This desirable administration is, of course, impractical. It would be more realistic to employ well designed controlled release drug delivery systems, where control of the drug blood level depends mainly upon the dose and the dosing interval (τ). This τ value has a strong influence on the ratio of maximum to minimum drug blood level, or in other words: the extent of fluctuations of drug levels in the biological fluid.

The relationship between τ, the fluctuations of the drug in the blood, and the elimination half-life time, $t_{1/2}$, have been best demonstrated by Theeuwes and Bayne [10]:

$$\tau \leqq \frac{t_{1/2}(\ln C_{max}/C_{min})}{\ln 2} . \tag{4}$$

When the ratio of C_{max} to C_{min} is 2, the dosing interval, τ, should be maximally equal to the elimination half-life time of the drug. Thus, low values, i.e., less then 2, for the C_{max}/C_{min} ratio and $t_{1/2}$ values less then 12, justify a controlled release dosage form for a drug.

The relationship between in-vitro and in-vivo data. The relation between the therapeutic effect of a drug as influenced by its absorption rate, and the *in-vitro* and/or *in-vivo* delivery rate of that drug, is controversial. Attempts to link these parameters have been described in the literature for the past twenty years [11,12]. Recently, Theeuwes described a model in which he distinguished two cases [13]:

a. The release rate of the dosage form is equal *in vitro* and *in vivo*:

$$k_{absorption} = F \cdot k_{in\text{-}vitro} \tag{5}$$

where: $k_{absorption}$ is the rate of drug absorption to the body, $k_{in\text{-}vitro}$ is the release rate of the dosage form as measured *in-vitro*, and F is a proportionality factor, expressed either as an amount (F_m), or rate (F_r), and for purposes of general discussion are assumed equal.

b. The release rates of the dosage form differ *in-vitro* and *in-vivo*.

$$K_{absorption} = F \cdot Q \cdot K_{in\text{-}vitro} \tag{6}$$

where $K_{absorption}$, $K_{in\text{-}vitro}$ and F are as defined in Eq. (4) and Q is a factor depending upon sensitivity of the *in-vivo* release rate to mechanism, structure, boundary condition changes and the change in magnitude from *in-vitro* to *in-vivo* conditions.

2.2 Localization Considerations

Drug targeting has been defined as selective *delivery* of a therapeutic agent to its site of action. The site of action, or target, can be a cell receptor, an enzyme, or other macromolecule. The delivery system in this case is achieved by coupling the drug to a carrier. The coupling can be physical in which case the drug is physically placed in a microencapsulated particle such as a liposome that will be recognized and bound to a desired site, or by covalently linking the drug to a molecule.

Assuming that particle size of the drug-carrier allows free passage through the vascular bed from the site of administration to the target cell or tissue, successful targetting depends also upon the ability of the drug-carrier complex to pass through other biological barriers. While passing these barriers the drug carrier linkage must remain intact and the system should avoid endocytosis to non-targetted site [14,15]. In an excellent review, Poznansky and Juliano have pointed out the following barriers that are typically encountered by the drug-carrier complex [16]:

1. The blood barrier: since it perfuses most areas of the body the blood is a tissue which is commonly used as a carrier. However, when foreign substances, such as drug delivery systems are placed into the blood, blood constituents quickly bind to these unrecognized substances in order to inactivate them as soon as possible, usually in enzymatic fashion.
2. The endothelial barrier of the capillary: a layer of endothelial cells which demarcate the vascular system and the tissue. This barrier permits passage of of macromolecules with a diameter of up to 30 nm by a process known as "transcytosis", but prevents the passage of larger particles like liposomes and most microspheres which therefore remain on the luminal side of the capillary endothelium [15,17].
3. The reticuloendothelial system barrier: a widespread system of cells which are mononuclear and phagocytic in nature that are considered to be macrophages. Their function is to remove foreign matter, such as macromolecules and microparticulate drug-carriers (liposome, microspheres) from the blood stream [18–20].
4. Cellular barriers: intracellular macromolecules and membrane organelles may inhibit the ability of drugs to react with the appropriate receptor and achieve a desired pharmacological response, by preventing internalized once they bind to the cell surface, or by internalization and then inactivation [16].

The ability to successfully pass through these barriers is a prerequisite for success of physical drug delivery systems such as liposomes, microspheres and nanocapsules. It should be noted that, other non-specific delivery systems are sometimes considered to be targeted systems, and it is not clear whether their accumulation in a tissue is a result of uptake by the reticuloendothelial system or specific uptake by the target cell due to proper drug delivery characteristics. Furthermore it is often not clear whether the desired activity is achieved by the ability of the drug-carrier complex to attach to a cell-specific site (receptor), or because of slower excretion of drug from the body [21].

A discussion of drug targetting systems will be presented in Section 3.

3 Strategies for Controlled Drug Delivery

3.1 Design Considerations

Achieving optimized, controlled drug therapy, involves successful interplay between the patient, the disease, the drug, and the drug delivery system. Some factors that should be taken into consideration are listed in Table 1 [22–25, 106]. While this brief listing of topics looks straightforward, a full review of each parameter for each drug candidate can save considerable expense and embarrassment. Thus, while at first glance it could appear that every drug could benefit by placement in a controlled drug delivery system, many of these drugs would be excluded from serious consideration by one or more of the factors listed in Table 1.

Table 1. Variables to be considered when designing controlled release drug Delivery systems

Variable	Possible constraint
1. *Drug Characteristics*	
a) *Physicochemical:*	
Dose size	— one Gm upper limit for single dose size. Should avoid unacceptably large volume
Aqueous solubility	— sparingly water soluble drugs are inherently sustained. Drug release to the biological fluids is controlled by dissolution — very water soluble useful for diffusion control
Drug pKa	— pH dependent solubility can restrict availability at absorption site — variable oral absorption due to regional pH differences in the GI tract
Partition coefficient	— desirable o/w partition coefficient is commonly 1000:1. Drugs with too high or too low a partition coefficient create tissue flux problems — route of administration should be carefully chosen in accordance with drug's partition coefficient
Charge	— may reduce absorption rate in GI tract, — may reduce membrane permeation, — formulation interactions with charged species
Molecular size	— good tissue permeability up to approximate m.w. of 500 to 1000. Larger molecules may also be difficult to formulate into controlled release drug delivery system
Stability	— unstable drugs may limit their use in some sustained relese-dosage forms and route of administration, e.g., hydrolytic instability and the oral route, or duration of contact with metabolic enzymes, e.g., peptidase
b) *Pharmacokinetics*	
Elimination half-life	— optimal $t_{1/2}$ for drug intended to be formulated as an oral sustained release form is 4–12 hours
Therapeutic Index	— drug with small therapeutic index requires presision of drug release control

Table 1. (continued)

Variable	Possible Constraint
Absorption	— slow absorption may limit the availability of drug, thus limit the use of controlled release drug delivery
	— regional absorption, e.g., upper part of the intestine in oral dosage, or specific absorption site may limit the use of controlled release dosage forms
Drug blood levels fluctuations	— C_{max}/C_{min} ratio should be no greater then the therapeutic index
2. *Physiological Factors*	
Age and sex	— newborn has immature hepatic and renal functions, influencing the ADME parameters
	— advanced age may decrease clearance function, reflected by increasing $t_{1/2}$ elimination — gastric emptying may be affected by age — patient compliance decreases with increasing age — more or less biological response to drug
GI motility	— under fasting conditions the gastro-ileal transit time may be 4–6 hours — under fed conditions gastro-ileal transit time is 6–9 hours — under fed conditions the gastric residence time is influenced by dosage form size
Circadian rhythm	— change in physiological process, on a daily basis, necessitating more or less drug
3. *Pathological Factors*	
Renal Diseases	— drug accumulation in the body when the kidney is the main clearing organ
Liver Diseases	— change in drug's volume of distribution and rate of metabolism
General Pathology	— increase or decrease barrier properties of drug reaching ther biophase, e.g., inflammed skin
4. *Patient Characteristics*	
Acute or Chronic Therapy	— route of administration
	— type of dosage form, e.g., in chronic treatment immediate fraction cannot be included — increase or decrease in biological response due to metabolizing enzyme induction or inhibition
Response to Drug	— some patients may be "fragile" in their response to drugs, i.e., a much more narrow therapeutic range
Ambulatory or bedridden	— route of administration,
	— changes in ADME parameters as a result of changes in physiological processes, e.g., blood flow, stomach emptying
Prophylaxis or treatment	— route of administration, — drug type and dose

3.2 Fabrication Strategies

The strategy to fabricate a controlled release dosage forms can involve several approaches, all aimed at achieving controlled drug therapy either by temporal control or spatial placement. Selected approaches are detailed below:

3.2.1 Physico-Chemical Approaches

a) Dissolution

The most common method to control drug release from a delivery system is by dissolution. Drugs that possess poor dissolution properties are inherently sustained since their dissolution rate is slower than subsequent absorption. Drugs that are highly water soluble can be converted to less soluble forms either by salt or derivative formation. A more common method is to incorporate the drug into either a nondegradable or biodegradable bead (matrix) where drug dissolution through the bead in the first case, or matrix dissolution in the second, determines drug availability. The dissolution process can be described by:

$$dc/dt = k_d A(C_s - C) \qquad (7)$$

Where dc/dt is the dissolution rate, k_d is the dissolution rate constant, A is the surface area of the particle undergoing dissolution, C_s is the aqueous saturation solubility of the drug, and C is the drug concentration in the bulk of the solution [26]. A constant dissolution rate is obtained as long as the right hand of Eq. (7) is held constant, i.e. constant surface area is maintained and excess drug yields a constant value for $(C_s - C)$ under sink conditions. Constant area dissolution systems are available only in some chemical reactions and it is normally difficult to maintain the surface area constant during dissolution, thus non-zero conditions commonly prevail. For spherical particles undergoing a change in their surface area while dissolving, the cube root Equation [27, 28] can be used:

$$W_0^{1/3} - W^{1/3} = kt \qquad (8)$$

Where W_0 is the initial weight of material, W is the weight of material left at time of measurement (t) and k is the cube root dissolution rate constant.

Most of the delivery systems utilizing dissolution to control drug release, employ poorly water soluble drugs or drug derivatives. Sometimes matrix formulations can be used for dissolution rate control, and some sophistication of these systems can be achieved by using matrix materials or polymers with pH or enzyme dependent dissolution [29]. Parenteral dissolution controlled dosage forms, have employed microspheres, nanoparticles or implants composed of biodegradable materials into which active drug is embedded. In order for these systems to perform as expected, it is necessary for them to be biocompatible at the injection site.

b) Diffusion

Diffusion is perhaps the most attractive mechanism for controlled drug delivery, primarily because with proper construction of the system a constant rate of drug release can be achieved. Basically, diffusion entails the movement of a molecule from a region of high to low concentration. The flux of drug, amount per area-time, across a membrane is defined by Fick's first law and can be written in steady state conditions as follows [30]:

$$J = -D(\Delta C/l) \tag{9}$$

Where D is the diffusion coefficient and ΔC is the concentration difference across a memrane of thickness l.

A form of Eq. (9) that permits conceptualization is:

$$\frac{dc}{dt} = \frac{DA}{l} \cdot (C_s - C) \tag{10}$$

where the above terms have been previously defined.

As in the case represented by Eq. (7), maintaining the terms on the right hand side of Eq. (10) constant, i.e., constant diffusion coefficient, surface area, and diffusional pathlength, with excess drug in the dosage-form so that $C_s - C \cong C_s$, generates a constant rate of drug release, i.e., $dc/dt = k$.

One can picture a water insoluble polymeric membrane surrounding drug particles. Drug release is governed by diffusion of the drug through the polymer film. As long as the polymer does not swell or disintegrate, a constant rate of drug release is expected.

Nondisintegrating matrix devices, represent an alternative type of diffusional systems. These matrices contain dissolved drug in the case of homogeneous matrices or dispersed drug in the case of heterogeneous matrices. Drug release by solvent elution is commonly characterized by an increasing diffusional pathlength i.e., non-zero order conditions. The appropriate Equation describing drug release from this type of system is presented below for a heterogeneous matrix [31]:

$$Q = [DE/\tau(2A - EC_S)\, C_S t]^{1/2} \tag{11}$$

Where Q is the weight of the drug released per surface are unit at time t, D is the diffusion coefficient of the drug in the solute, E is the porosity of the matrix, τ is a tortuosity

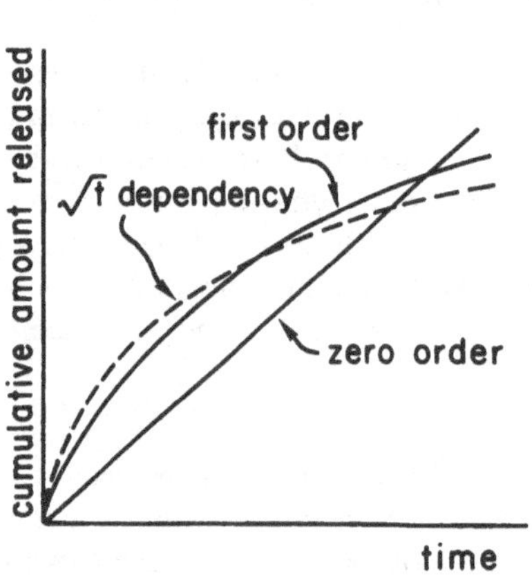

Fig. 2. Pictorial scheme of three types of kinetic profiles representing zero-order drug release, first-order drug release and $\sqrt{t}$ dependent drug release

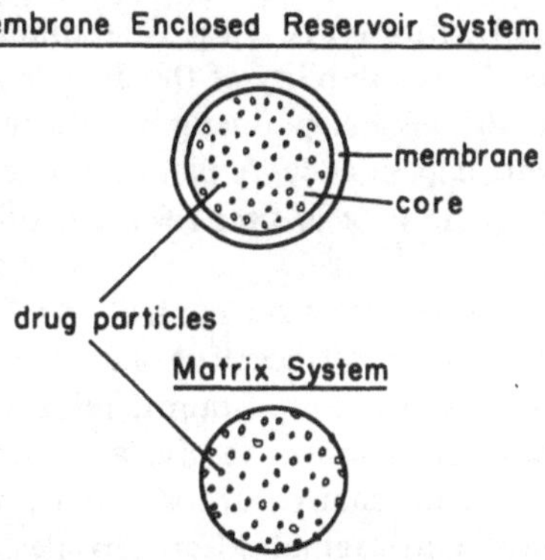

Fig. 3. Pictorial scheme of two controlled release dosage forms based on the diffusion principle (drug can be dispersed or dissolved in the system). Note the existence of drug particles at the surface area of the matrix system, causing a relatively high rate at the beginning of the drug release procedure

Table 2. Some examples for diffusion-controlled reservoir, and diffusion-controlled matrix devices [23)]

Diffusion-Controlled Reservoir Devices		
Drug	*Coating Material*	*Dosage Form*
Cyclazocine	DL-polylactic acid	Microcapsules dispersed in sesame oil for injection
Clofibrate	Gelatin	Microcapsules
Caffeine, salicylic Acid	Ethylcellulose	Film strips
Progesterone	Polyhydroxymethacrylate	Film strips
Potassium chloride	Polymethylmethacrylate, polyethylene glycol 600, polystyrene, various waxes	Radiation-polymerized beads
Methapyridene, pentobarbital, salicylic acid	Hydroxypropyl cellulose-polyvinyl acetate	Film strips
Salicylic acid, caffeine, tripelennamide	Polyethylene glycol-ethylcellulose	Film strips
Diffusion-Controlled Matrix Devices		
Tripelennamine HCl	Carnauba wax, stearyl alcohol	Granules compressed into cores
Morphine sulphate	Silicone	Spherical pellets
Sulfaethylthiadiazole	Glyceryl tristearate	Particles
Sodium pentobarbital, methapyrilene HCl, ephedrine HCl, dextromethorphane HBr	Methylacrylate-methyl methacrylate	Tablets
Sodium salicylate	Polyvinyl chloride polyethylene halogenated fluorocarbon	Tablets
Sulfanilamide, caffeine, potassium acid phthalate	Polyethylene	Tablets
Chlorpheniramine maleate	Hydrated methylcellulose	Tablets
Nicotinic acid, quinidine sulphate, antihistamines	Hydroxypropylmethyl-cellulose, sodium carboxy-methylcellulose	Tablets
Phenylpropanolamine	Wax-fatty acid mixture	Tablets

factor, a term to account for a complex diffusional pathway, A is the total amount of drug present in the matrix per unit volume, and C_S is solubility of the drug in the solute. In this case, because of the non-constant diffusional pathlength, release of drug is not zero-order but has a square root of time dependency. A pictorial scheme demonstrating typical zero-order, first-order and square root of time release profiles on a linear scale, are represented in Fig. 2.

The most common application of diffusion for release rate control involves membrane coated tablets and microcapsules. However, more recent devices such as the Ocusert® which is an intraocular drug delivery system for sustained release of pilocarpine to the eye, or transdermal patches, have been shown to give a constant rate of drug delivery. Coated tablets are widely used for many purposes and for a variety of routes of administration, e.g., oral, buccal, and vaginal. Microcapsules, or nanocapsules can serve as micropolymeric devices to control drug release for specialized application, e.g., for drug delivery to the eye or parenterally to deliver vaccine in a modulated fashion [32]. Figure 3 describes schematically the difference between drug delivery systems designed as diffusion-controlled reservoir and diffusion-controlled matrix devices. Table 2 summarizes some examples for drugs and materials used to coat or to form matrices that have been published lately [23].

c) Osmosis

Drug delivery systems based on osmotic pressure were developed by Alza and described extensively by Theeuwes [33]. The osmotic tablet consists of a core of drug and, in most cases, additional agent to assist in creating osmotic pressure, both coated with a semipermeable membrane. The membrane permits an eluting solvent such as water to penetrate into the tablet and generate an osmotic pressure, but does not permit movement of drug or electrolyte. An orifice in the coat allows the drug solution to be pumped out at a rate equal to the solvent volume uptake rate. As long as excess electrolyte and drug remains in the tablet, a constant release rate is maintained. Once the concentration of the osmotic agent falls below saturation the release rate decreases in a first order fashion. Thus, the rate of drug delivery from the osmotic pump is controlled by the rate of water absorption into the device, as represented by the following Equation:

$$\frac{dV}{dt} = \frac{KA}{l}(\Delta\pi - \Delta P) \tag{12}$$

Here, dv/dt is the solvent flow rate, K is the membrane permeability constant, A is the membrane surface area, l is the membrane thickness, $\Delta\pi$ is the osmotic pressure difference, and ΔP is the hydrostatic pressure difference. When $\Delta\pi >> \Delta P$, Equation (12) can be reduced to:

$$\frac{dV}{dt} = \frac{KA}{l} \cdot \Delta\pi \tag{13}$$

Thus, when A, l, and $\Delta\pi$ are maintained constant for a particular polymeric membrane enclosing excess electrolyte, a constant, i.e., zero-order delivery rate is achieved:

$$dv/dt = k` \tag{14}$$

This system is essentially independent of pH, stirring rate effects, and other environmental influences. The only commercial example of the system is the phenylpropanolamine product Acutrim®.

d) Ion Exchange

These systems are based on positively or negatively charged drugs which form salts to charged polymeric resins. Cationic exchangers use groups such as SO_3^-, $COO^=$ and $PO_3^=$, and anionic exchangers use amino groups such as NH_3^+, NH_2^+ and N^+.

When orally administered, the system exchanges drug with appropriate counter ions in the Gl tract. Representative drug release from the system is as shown below [34]:

In the stomach:

$$\text{Resin} - SO_3^- NH_3^+ - \text{Drug} + H^+ \rightleftharpoons \text{Resin} - SO_3H + H + \text{Drug} - NH_3$$
$$\text{Resin} - NH_3^+ OOC^- - \text{Drug} + Cl^- \rightleftharpoons \text{Resin} - NH_3^+ Cl^- + \text{Drug}$$

In the intestine:

$$\text{Resin} - SO_3^- NH_3^+ - \text{Drug} + NaCl \rightleftharpoons \text{Resin} - SO_3^- NA^+ + \text{Drug} - NH_3^+ Cl^-$$
$$\text{Resin} - NH_3^+ OOC^- - \text{Drug} + NaCl \rightleftharpoons \text{Resin} - NH_3^+ Cl^- + \text{Drug} - COO^- Na^+$$

Table 3. Examples of controlled release dosage forms using drug-resin complex to control drug release [34]

Therapeutic Category	Brand Name	Drug
Sympathomimetics	Asmapax®	Ephedrine
	Dexten®	Dexamphetamine
	Mirapront®	Phentermine
	Duromin®	Phentermine
Antitussives	Longatin®	Noscapine
	Histionex®	Phenyltoloxamine
	Tussionex®	Hydrokodon
	Codipront®	Codeine
Antihistaminics		Dextromethorphan
		Methapyrilene, carbinoxamine, chlorpheniramine, diphenhydramine, promethazine, pyrilamine, tripelennamine, pyribenzamine
Anticholinergics	Spartipax®	Atropine
		Homatropine, scopolamine, methscopolamine bromide, trihexyphenidyl HCl, diphemanil methyl sulphate
Antelmintics		Piperazine, levamisol
Antibacterial		Neomycin, sulfadiazine, penicilline V and G
Others		Morphine, gentisic acid, salycylic acid, quinine

The release rate of these systems can be further modified by coating the drug-resin complex with a rate limiting polymer. By mixing various ratios of coated and uncoated drug-resin, the rate of release can be regulated. As an example, this technique has been used with phenylpropanolamine to yield a twice daily controlled release drug delivery system [35]. Table 3 summarizes a list of products using the technique of drug-resin combination to control drug release.

e) Liquid Systems

Liquid sustained/controlled release drug-delivery systems are usually difficult to prepare, especially oral products, since an aqueous based vehicle is required for their manufacture, and, unless one starts with an aqueous drug suspension where a saturated solution is already present, upon storage the drug can leach out, giving a potentially hazardous dose.

Ion exchange resins, with or without a barrier polymeric coating, have been used in liquid products for a variety of charged drugs to overcome this shelf-like problem. Since release of drug requires the presence of a suitable exchange ion, the presence of water as such has no theoretical effect on drug release.

Lately, multiple emulsions i.e., drug emulsified in a hydrophobic phase which in turn is emulsified once again in water, have been tested as oral controlled relase dosage forms [36]. To date there are no commercial products employing this approach, but, provided the emulsion remains intact in the route of administration, the potential of this system is obvious.

The most common use of liquid sustained release products is for parenteral administration of drugs. The following systems are used in the design and fabrication of liquid parenteral controlled release dosage forms: (1) aqueous suspensions, (2) oily solutions, (3) oily suspensions, (4) emulsions, (5) aqueous dispersions of microcapsules, nanocapsules, microspheres, or liposomes. The rate of drug release out of the first three systems is often decreased by adding viscosity inducing agent such as metallic stearates, or metallic salts of other fatty acids.

1. *Aqueous suspensions*: The mean dissolution rate dM/dt of solid particles in an aqueous suspension of specified viscosity is described by Eq. (15) and shown illustratively in Fig. 4 [26]:

$$\frac{dM}{dt} = \frac{k \cdot T}{6\pi\eta r} \cdot \frac{C_S}{l} \cdot \frac{K}{R} \tag{15}$$

where k is the Boltzman constant, T is the absolute temperature, r is the hydrodynamic radius of the drug molecule, η is the viscosity of the aqueous medium, C_S is the saturation solubility of the drug, l is the thickness of the diffusion layer, R is the drug particle radius and K is a constant.

From Eq. (15) it is clear that the mean dissolution rate decreases when the suspension viscosity increases and the drug particle radius increases. It is this Equation, that enables calculation of the release rate of a drug after addition of viscosity inducing agents like methylcellulose to parenteral suspensions. There is an optimum ratio of viscosity to particle size that permits syringability, minimum settling of particles and yet a usable dissolution rate. The desirable ratio between solid and liquid phases in injectable suspensions is 1:200 to 1:20 [37], and the optimal solid particle size should be below 10 micrometer [38].

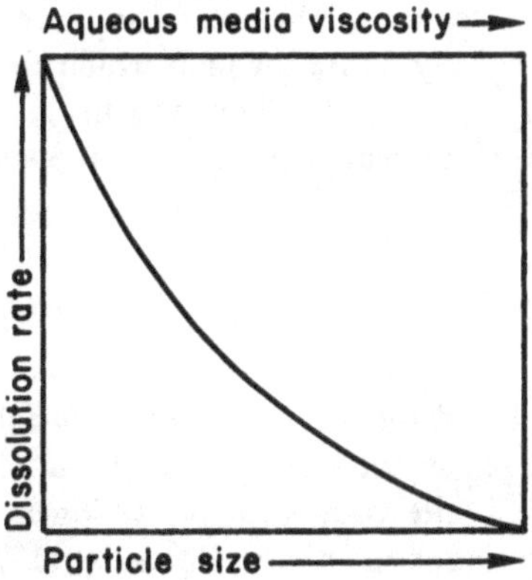

Fig. 4. Schematic representation of the influence of aqueous phase viscosity and drug particle size on dissolution rate of aqueous suspensions

A fundamental, but poorly understood, aspect of parenterally administered controlled drug delivery systems is biocompatiblity of the system at the injection site. Inflammation, protective isolation of the injected mass and invasion of inflammatory substances at the injection site can have a profound influence on drug release and hence drug performance. This is particularly true for parenterally administered peptides/proteins where the invasion of macrophages and proteases can inactivate the drug and substantially alter the release rate of drug from the dosage form [39].

2. *Oily solutions*: The fraction of drug that is available for absorption from an oily solution is governed by two factors:

— the drug's partition coefficient
— the phase volume ratio of the oily phase to the aqueous phase in the tissue.

A general Equation describing the fractional concentration of a drug in the aqueous phase (f) is as follows:

$$f = \frac{1 + \alpha}{1 + K\alpha} \tag{16}$$

Where α is the volume ratio of oil to water (V_0/V_w), and K is the ratio of drug concentrations in the oil and aqueous phases (D_0/D_w).

The fraction of drug in each phase remains constant as long as the ratio of aqueous/oily phases does not change. In the body the entire aqueous phase is a physiological parameter and hence considered to be constant. Therefore under physiological conditions, changes in the aqueous/oil phase ratio are governed mainly by the volume of the oil phase, and thus the relationship of drug/oil phase is of a great importance.

The rate of drug release from the oil can be modified by addition of viscosity inducing agents, e.g., incorporating aluminium salt of fatty acid to the oil, causing it to gel and hence reducing drug release rate due to two different mechanisms: minimizing the surface area at the site of injection, and reducing the diffusion rate of drug molecule through the oil [40].

Emulsions: Modelling of emulsions is more difficult since three phases are involved: the aqueous phase in which the drug is dissolved, and oily phase through which the drug must pass, and the physiological aqueous phase through which the drug is absorbed. A representive equation describing the fraction of drug that is in the aqueous physiological fluid (f_1) after administration is:

$$f_1 = \frac{1 + V_2/V_1 + V_0/V_1}{1 + (V_0/V_1)\,K_1 + (V_2/V_1)\,(K_1/K_2)} \qquad (17)$$

where K_1 is the partition coefficient between the oil and the aqueous physiological phase, K_2 is the partition coefficient between the oil phase and the aqueous phase of the emulsion, V_0 is the volume of the oil phase, V_1 is the volume of physiological aqueous phase, and V_2 is the volume of the emulsion aqueous phase. Equation (17) can be simplified by the following assumptions: usually K_1 and K_2 are about equal, and $V_1 >> V_2$, so $V_2/V_1 \cong 0$. This Equation can now be written as follows:

$$f_1 = \frac{1 + V_0/V_1}{1 + (V_0/V_1)\,K_1} = \frac{1 + \alpha}{1 + K_1\alpha} \qquad (18)$$

Equation (18) is identical to Eq. (16) and therefore it can be seen that there is no advantage in using 0/W emulsions rather than oily solutions. Table 4 summarizes some depot parenteral dosage forms [41].

Table 4. Some examples of injectable depot products [41]

Drug	Brand Name	Type of Preparation
Procaine penicilline G' suspension,	Duracillin® (Lilly) Wycillin® (Wyeth)	Thixotropic aqueous suspension
Cyanocobalamine zinc tannate suspension,	Depinar® (Armour)	A mixture of tannate salt together with soluble Vit. B_{12}, suspended in sesame oil
Medroxyprogesterone acetate suspension,	Depo-Provera® (Upjohn)	Aqueous suspension
Fluphenazinc enanthate and decanoate,	Prolixin Enanthate® Prolixin Decanoate® (Squibb)	Bioerodible ester in oil solution
ACTH zinc tannate/gelatin,	H.P. Acthar® (Armour)	ACTH in 16% gelatin aqeous solution
Microcrystalline desoxycorticosterone pivalate,	Percorten Pivaltate® (Ciba)	Oleaginous suspension
Testosterone enanthate/ estradiol valerate,	Ditate-ds® (Savage)	Solution in ethyl oleate
Nandrolone decanoate	Deca Durabolin® (Organon)	Bioerodible ester
Insulin-zinc suspension	Ultralente® (Lente) Semi-Lente® (Novo)	Aqueous suspension of insulin with $ZnCl_2$

3.2.2 Mechanical Approach

This approach is commonly used when a clinical situation demands a therapeutic approach not easily satisfied through conventional menas, e.g., when a large drug quantity over an extended time period is beyond the capability of conventional controlled release formulation and an external or implantable pump would therefore be indicated. Mechanical delivery of drug through an external or implanted pump is becoming increasingly popular due, in part, to miniaturization of the system and reliability of the delivery rate. Whereas in the not-too-distant past, such pump delivery of drug would have been largely restricted to hospitalized patients, there is an increasing use in the ambulatory outpatient population.

a) External pumps

Portable external pumps appeared in the beginning of the 1970's, in the treatment of diabetes mellitus. Such pumps claimed to have better control over blood insulin levels than conventional therapeutic treatment of several daily injections [6,42]. These insulin delivery units were composed of a syringe which controlled insulin levels by varying the interval between pulses ("syringe pumps"), or peristaltic or piston pumps which controlled the rate of insulin supply on a continuous basis. These pumps generally supply two distincts rates of insulin delivery to provide the patients basal and prandial needs.

b) Implantable Pumps

The ideal implantable pump should posses the following characteristics [43]:

Performance: It is expected that the pump should be sufficiently flexible to provide a wide range of drug release rates, dictated by a variety of clinical situations. Reliable and accurate drug delivery over long time periods are of importance in order to justify the minor surgery associated with implantation (the usual demand is 2–5 years).
Safety: The pump should be biocompatible and should not release toxic, antigenic, mutagenic or carcinogenic materials into the surrounding tissues.
Convenience of use: The drug reservoir and the energy source, e.g. battery, must be easy to refill or replace. Ease of programming is also highly desirable.
Sterilizability: The usual way of sterilizing implantable devices is by irradiation. Care should be taken to avoid incompatibilities of the sterilization procedure with the device components, including the drug.
Applications of implantable pumps: Implantable pumps are mainly used to control insulin blood levels in treatment of diabetes, in what is now known as closed-loop, i.e., self-monitored, and open-loop, i.e., constant administration without regulation devices. It is worth noting that the advantage of this kind of administration is limited to compliant patients and has not been established to be superior to multiple intramuscular injections, among young or non-compliant patients [6,44,45]. Implantable pumps have also been used in cancer chemotherapy; success has been reported in the treatment of colorectal cancer that had metastasized to the liver and in the treatment of central nervous system tumors [46,47]. Systemic administration of heparin using implantable osmotic pumps for the treatment of severe thromboembolic disease that is refractory to treatment with oral anticoagulants or antiplatelet drugs, has been reported [48,49].

c) Osmotic Minipumps

Systems that rely on osmotic pressure to deliver drugs have been described earlier. Such systems can be modified for implant purposes and a typical commercial example is the Alzet®, an implantable osmotic minipump used extensively in animal investigations. Another technique uses the combination of flourocarbon propellent and body heat as a driving force for drug release. In Infusaid®, vapor pressure, forces drug solution through a flow regulator at a constant rate [50]. Basically, one can either implant the entire pump, which is not commonly done, or simply localize a fine tube from the pump to some desired location.

3.2.3 Prodrugs/Analog Approach

Two approaches can be used to chemically modify the delivery of drug. In the first case a molecular modification is used to produce a new drug entity with similar pharmacological properties, i.e., an *analog*, where in the second a functional group is attached to the drug molecule to produce an inactive compound, i.e., a *prodrug*. In the body fluids, the prodrug is converted back to the original drug and an inactive molecule [51]. Two goals can potentially be achieved by using a well-designed prodrug to control drug delivery: (a) systemic drug action will be sustained, (b) targeting to a desired organ is possible.

a. The first goal can be achieved in either of two ways: extending the absorptive phase, i.e. the prodrug will be absorbed at a slower rate than the parent drug, or by sustaining the degradation rate of the prodrug to the drug molecule once it is in the biological system. When using a prodrug it is generally not possible to

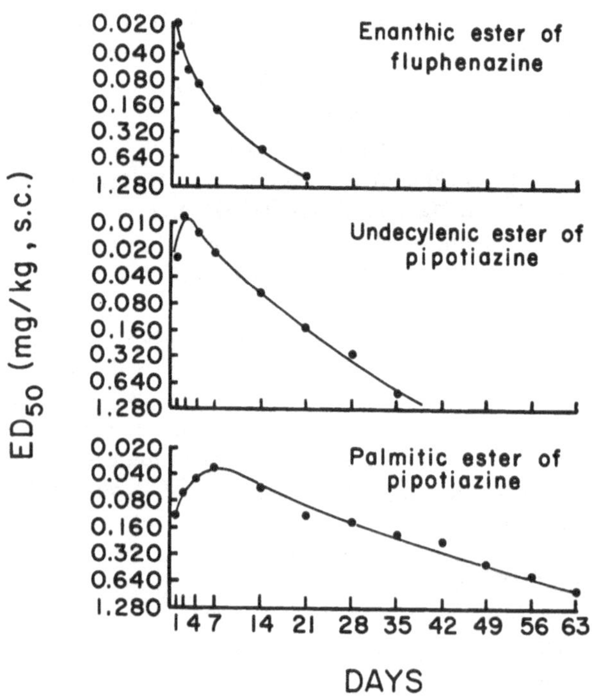

Fig. 5. Antiapomorphine activity as expressed by ED_{50} as a function of time in dog, caused by enanthic ester of fluphenazine, undecylenic ester of pipotiazine, and palmitic ester of pipotiazine [53]

control its pharmacological effect once at the receptor site, thus the advantage of the analog approach. By using the appropriate analog, one can regulate and control its elimination rate, and hence, achieve sustained action.

A typical example of the prodrug approach in the design of sustained release drug derivatives is with steroids. The early use of these drugs was characterized by low absorption and fast metabolism and excretion. Methods of slowing their duration of activity included synthesis of long chain fatty acid esters and derivatives sterically hindered at or near the site of hydrolysis [52]. A clear demonstration of how the duration of activity of a drug can be altered by using the prodrug approach is shown in Fig. 5 [53]. The elimination half-life of the ester derivative of pipotiazine is increased by increasing the chain length of the ester. Valpromide, the primary amide of valproic acid, is recognized as a prodrug for valproic acid [54, 55] although it is used for a different therapeutic purpose. Recently it was formulated as a sustained release prodrug of valproic acid [56].

b. Stella and Himmelstein have summarized the proper strategy to achieve successful targeting via the prodrug approach [14]. The steps in the strategy are outlined as follows: (1) identify the biochemical pathway of the disease; (2) definite the organ (or cell) demanding therapeutic involvement, including transit barriers; (3) study the entire organ properties that could be utilized to help effect targetting, such as membrane transport or surface properties; (4) select a drug that is effective at the receptor level, but based on physical/chemical properties, is limited in its ability to reach its site of action; (5) modify the drug candidate so that when the prodrug reaches the active site it will release the active drug.

It should be noted that the prodrug approach is the complete opposite of the "soft" drug approach. "Soft" drugs are defined as drugs which undergo predictable and controllable metabolism to non-toxic moieties, after they have elicited their pharmacological response, in contrast to "hard" drugs, which do not undergo metabolism [57]. While prodrugs are entities that transform themselves to the parent drugs, soft drugs do not change before acting unless a predetermined metabolic procedure is involved.

3.2.4 Drug Targetting

Figure 6 schematically represents two ways of targeting drug to the cell with the aid of a drug-carrier. In the first one, drug is separated from its carrier in front of the cell membrane and the drug penetrates by simple diffusion. Alternatively, drug is internalized while still bound to its carrier by means of pinocytosis or phagocytosis. In the cell it acts either free or in complexed form [58].

The major criteria of a carrier-drug complex has been detailed earlier. Stella and Himmelstein, while discussing targetting via prodrugs, have pointed out three factors necessary for successful targetting [14]:

a. Ready transport of a drug to its target site, and subsequent rapid uptake.
b. Selective cleavage of a carrier-drug complex to the active drug at the target organ.
c. Succesfull retention of drug by the target organ.

Some targetted delivery systems are described below:

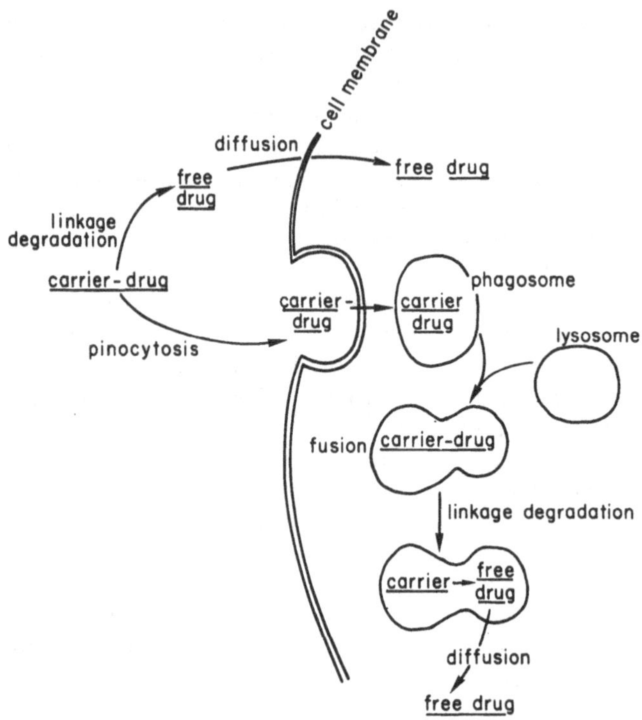

Fig. 6. Schematic representation of several pathways for drug to penetrate the cell [58]

a) Particulate Systems

Under this broad terminology one finds drug delivery systems such as micro — and nano encapsulated drugs, and small particle matrix systems. There are two ways to distinguish between these systems: (1) by mechanism of drug loading, e.g., entrapping the drug as a solid or liquid core by the carrier walls, e.g., microcapsules and nano-capsules, or embeding the drug in a carrier matrix, e.g., microspheres and polymeric beads, (2) by particle size (see Table 5).

By definition, particulate systems are less specific than others, mainly because of their restricted passage through the capillary endothelial barrier. Therefore the main organs are the liver, spleen or lungs. Targetting in this connection relates to the entrapment process of the particles in the reticuloendothelial system. Once the particles have arrived at their target, release of drug is controlled by one of the following mechanism: (1) bioerosion of the wall or matrix with subsequent release of drug, (2) diffusion of drug through the wall or out of the matrix, or (3) endocytosis into the tissue. Indeed many particulate systems containing anti-tumor agents are designed to release the entrapped drug by diffusion [59,60].

b) Liposomes

Liposomes are phospholipids that, after being dispersed in water, form spherical structures containing aqueous layers surrounded by phospholipid bilayer membranes [14,61]. Besides being a useful model to study membrane behavior they can serve

Table 5. Some carriers used for drug targetting [21]

Carrier type	*Particle diameter*	*Release controlled by:*
Microcapsule (with core and wall)	1–1000 μm	— Concentration of drug in core; — polymer wall thickness; — diffusivity of drug in polymer; — solubility of drug in polymer; — biodegradability or bioerodibility of system
Microsphere (matrices)	0.2–100 μm	— concentration of drug in matrix; — diffusivity of drug in polymer; — solubility of drug in polymer; — biodegradibility or bioerodibility of system; — degree of crosslinking — thickness of diffusion layer
Macroemulsions	0.2–100 μm	— partition coefficient of drug; — metabolism of oily phase of
Microemulsions	40 nm	emulsion; stability in-vivo
Multilamellar liposomes (vesicles)	400–3500 nm	— adsorption of blood components; — diffusion of drug; — drug solubility; — nature of lipid comprising vesicle; — liposome-cell interaction;
Unilamellar	20–1000 nm	— molecular weight of drug; — partition coefficient of drug; — hydrolysis of phospholipid
Low density lipoprotein	24 nm	— cholesteryl ester exchange; — intracellular digestion
Macromolecular carrier (drug attached by electrostatic or covalent bonds)		— scission of linkage between drug and backbone; — nature of link between drug and carrier; — rate of uptake into cell; — molecular weight of carrier; — pH changes

as drug carriers, since water or lipid-soluble materials can be entrapped in the aqueous or the bilayer spaces. A large variety of drugs have been incorporated into liposomes in the last 10 years and include antitumor agents, polyene antibiotics, antibacterials, and antiparasitic drugs [62].

The advantage of liposomes in targetting is clearly illustrated by the following observations: (1) Recent investigations indicate that liposomes can provide efficient delivery of immunomodulating agents such as lymphokines, MDP, and C-reactive protein to macrophages in order to increase their ability to attack and destroy tumor cells [64–66]. (2) Liposomes can be used to reduce the toxicity of antitumor drugs like Adriamycin, by simply entrapping them until they reach the target organ [67]. Likewise, it was recently found that liposomal amphotericin-B is toxic to fungal cells but not to mammalian cells [68]. (3) Antimicrobial drugs that are found to be effective in vitro (aminoglycosides) can be used with liposomes as carriers to the intracellular compartment of macrophages [69].

Table 5 summarizes various particulate drug-carriers and their properties.

c) Resealed Erythrocytes

Red blood cells, if loaded with drugs, have potentially attractive features for drug delivery. The half-life of a normal red blood cell is approximately 30 days and thus they have effective circulation times of about 120 days. Morever, a surface modified red blood cell will be quickly sequestered by the reticuloendothelial system and thus specific targeting to these organs is possible.

One can achieve drug loading of red blood cells through electrical or osmotic means. In the first technique an electric discharge is passed through a suspension of red blood cells in which drug has been placed, causing the cell to open and exchange its contents with the bathing drug solution. The cells eventually close and entrap drug [70]. In the second technique, erythrocytes are suspended in a hypotonic medium, causing them to swell and enlarge their membrane pores, thus allowing drug solution to penetrate into the cell. Incubating the suspension in an isotonic solution at 37 °C reseals the pores.

Loaded red blood cells have been used primarily in enzyme replacement therapy [71]. The disadvantage of the method is that the sites of pathogenesis in enzyme deficiency are not readily accessible to erythrocytes or any microparticulate system.

Two major deficiencies of the drug loaded red blood cells are: (1) relatively low drug loading capacity, i.e., typically $< 10\%$, and (2) it is not yet possible to load the cells without some surface changes leading to rapid sequestration from the blood.

d) Monoclonal Antibodies

Targetting drugs using monoclonal antibodies as carriers is relatively new to drug delivery systems. These high affinity antibodies are superior to conventional antibodies (polyclonal) by providing a high level of specificity even when used at relatively high dilutions. A monoclonal antibody is synthesized by fusing an immunized lymphocyte together with a myeloma cell line to produce a hybridoma and then cloning it. The product is characterized by sequence homogenity that causes it to elicit high specifity, thus recognizing a single amino acid substitution in a protein [72].

The advantages of monoclonal antibodies over polyclonal antibodies are: (1) physico-chemical concepts like equilibrium, reaction rate, and diffusion rate constants can be quantitatively used in these systems; (2) reproducibility of product, allowing development of commercial products. (3) specifity can be designed by either production of antibodies with unique specificities at each of their functional domains, or by linking monoclonal antibodies with different specificities [73].

In spite of some successful reports about therapeutic treatment, primarily with antitumor agents such as methotrexate and adriamycin, and mostly with animal models, this technique is considered to be at an early stage. Problems such as immunogenicity and a lack of absolute means of purification [74], are perhaps some of the reasons for minimal therapeutic use but extensive application in analysis, i.e., immunoassays and in diagnostic kits.

e) Magnetic Fields as Targetting Tools

An interesting approach to targetting a carrier-drug complex to a specific organ is by incorporating magnetite (Fe_3O_4) in a drug delivery system and using an external magnetic field for system localization [75]. Impressive results were achieved by Yoshida in treating rat tumors, but the limitation of this technique restricts it to large, easily accessible tumors. An interesting application of this technique, for the purpose of controlled delivery of peptides and proteins has been reported by Langer and his group, using an oscillating magnetic field to reversibly increase, by up to 100%, the release rate of bovine serum albumin from an ethylene-vinyl acetate copolymer matrix containing magnetic steel beads [76].

4 Advances in Drug Delivery via Selected Routes of Administration

4.1 Localized Drug Delivery

Localized drug delivery can be broadly defined as regional delivery to specific areas of the body. These areas include various regions of the Gl tract, the nose, the eye, the vagina and the skin. The major parameters that influence performance of these systems are the degree of contact of the drug delivery system with the absorption site (membrane), and its ability to maintain contact [77].

Two localized drug delivery systems have been chosen to demonstrate this approach bioadhesive and transdermal systems.

4.1.1 Bioadhesion

Oral controlled release drug delivery systems are limited to some extent by (a) the relatively short gastrointestinal transit time for all dosage forms, and (b) the relative inability to maintain a drug delivery system at a particular site for an extend period of time. Thus, the duration of most orally administered systems is 8–12 hours and it is almost impossible to predetermine a specific region of the Gl tract in which drug absorption will be localized.

An attempt to affect Gl transit time by varying the density, size, or viscosity of the dosage-form particles was recently reported [78–80]. However, this collective influence was minimal in human subjects. An alternative approach is to use bioadhesives. A bioadhesive is a substance with the ability to attach to biological surfaces and is capable of being retained on that surface for an extended period of time [81,82].

Polymeric material that attaches to mucosal surfaces, referred to as mucoadhesives, can attach through both covalent and non-covalent means. Recent work has focused on non-covalent attachment and rather dramatic clinical reports on erodible bioadhesive system to treat carcinoma coli have been reported by Nagai and his group [83,84].

Extensive work by Peppas [85] and Robinson [81,82] to delineate mechanism(s) of attachment have also been reported. The intent of these mechanistic studies is to not only identify new classes of bioadhesive polymers but to achieve some degree of specificity of attachment. Thus, bacteria possess great specificity for adhering to various biological locations such as the large bowel at the Gl tract. It is a reasonable end point that a good understanding of the mechanism of polymeric adhesion and associated structure activity relations could lead to similar specificity.

Using bioadhesive polymers, together with sustained release dosage forms, can yield a once daily oral dosing product. The following drug properties are particularly amenable to bioadhesive formulation for oral use:

a. A narrow and specific "absorption window". It is expected that localization and successful adhesion in the absorptive area would improve bioavailability.
b. Limited absorption due to low pH dependent solubility or an active saturable process in the Gl tract.
c. Limited absorption due to Gl motility which removes these drugs from the proximal small intestine before absorption is completed, regardless of the mechanism of absorption.

In all cases slow gastric release of the drug may increase intestinal absorption efficiency and bioavailability [86, 87].

Bioadhesion in the Gl tract occurs to the mucous coating of the epithelium. Mucin contains more then 95% water and coats the entire gastrointestinal tract as well as the eye, the nasal, the cervical and vaginal cavities. Adhesion has been studied [81, 82, 88], with regard to attachment of a variety of bioadhesive polymers that can serve as platforms for drug delivery when in contact with the mucin layer.

A typical example of using a bioadhesive to achieve sustained release as well as to improve bioavailability of a drug has been demonstrated by Longer et al. [86], in which chlorothiazide was incorporated into cross-linked albumin beads, mixed with the bioadhesive, polycarbophil, and administered to rats. Bioavailability from the bioadhesive formulation was 1.95 times greater then from the regular sustained release formulation without the bioadhesive and the duration of the drug blood level was twice that in the bioadhesive as compared to the nonbioadhesive case as shown in Fig. 7.

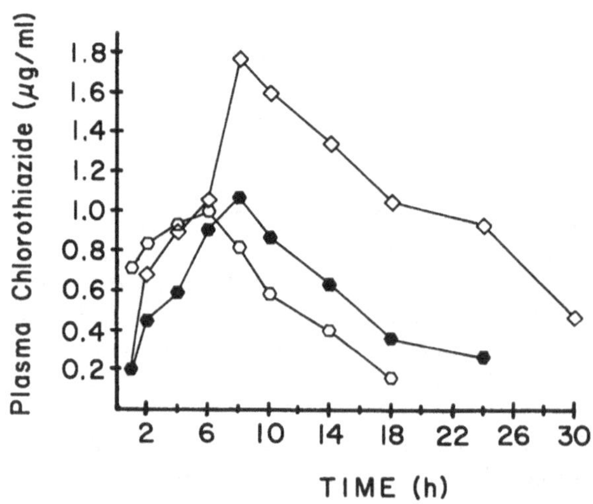

Fig. 7. Chlorothiazide plasma levels in rats after administering: 1. drug powder (○), 2. albumin beads containing drug (●), and 3, mixture of albumin beads containing drug with polycarbophil (◇) [86]

4.1.2 Transdermal Delivery Systems

Sustained delivery of drugs to the skin, either for a topical or systemic effect, is a relatively old approach, and products like steroid or alkaloidloaded tapes or plasters are well known. Newer approaches, including transdermal patches, allow considerable control over the release rate [77]. The potential benefits of transdermal drug delivery can be summarized as follows:

1. Improved patient compliance, especially in cases that require relatively frequent dosing of the same drug when administered orally, due to a limited residence time in the Gl tract.
2. Controlled level of drug in biological fluids, as well as relatively rapid drug input in some specific therapeutic situations.
3. Avoidance of hepatic-first-pass metabolism.

The main disadvantage of this type of delivery system is the significant barrier posed by the skin with corresponding restrictions on the total amount of drug that can be delivered per day using a 5–10 cm^2 surface area platform. At present, transdermal administration is effectively limited to relatively potent and lipophilic drugs [89].

For most of the presently marketed transdermal drugs, the skin is rate limiting in the transport process. Moreover, some commercial devices have little rate control over the availability of drug, relying instead on the natural resistance of the skin. These systems can present overdose problemsto those individuals with damaged skin and/or high skin permeability [90].

Typical drugs used in transdermal delivery systems are summarized in Table 6 [90,91]

Table 6. Drugs that are currently approved for transdermal delivery in the U.S.

Drug	*Therapeutic Duration in Transdermal Delivery*
Glyceryl Trinitrate	24 h
Scopolamine	72 h
Clonidine	1 week
Estradiol	[a]

[a] approval is expected in the near future

5 Evaluation of Controlled Drug Delivery

5.1 *In-Vitro Evaluation*

1. System Description

The primary purposes of the *in-vitro* test are: (1) to provide a development tool to evaluate and compare drug delivery systems in various stages of development, (2) to provide a meaningful quality control procedure to evaluate if the drug delivery system meets the requirement of a controlled rate of release for each lot of product.

There are a variety of dissolution tests all of which have evolved as a model of the human Gl tract. Thus, one uses aqueous media at pH 2 or 7.4, with or without enzymes, the apparatus itself creates turbulence by stirring or rotation. While these systems are considered to be satisfactory for immediate release dosage forms, they do not routinely correlate with *in-vivo* results for controlled release delivery systems.

The following elements are desirable for a successful *in-vitro* dissolution test:

a. An appropriate dissolution media that imitates as closely as possible the immediate environment in which the dosage form releases its drug. It is desirable to have a predetermined ratio between the volume of the dissolution medium and the final solubility of the drug, to insure sink conditions, an appropriate temperature, and the presence of enzymes, buffers or surfactants.
b. Appropriate dissolution apparatus with well defined hydrodynamics e.g., stirring, stirring rate and intensity of flow in the case of flow cells.

Many plain, as well as more complex systems have been developed using these guidelines [92,93], but indeed, there are as yet no compendial or other regulatory guidelines for dissolution tests of controlled release dosage forms.

2. Modeling

Mathematical modelling of drug release kinetics for a controlled release dosage form is necessary to predict experimental results and in this way minimize the number of experiments, as well as understand the physical mechanisms of release by comparing the kinetic data to mathematical models [94]. It should be pointed out that the enormous variety of drug delivery systems that possess different release rate characteristics makes it almost impossible to develop one, or even several, general mathematical models, that will be specific enough to identify, and characterize all parameters simultaneously. For general, practicle purposes, Eqs. (8, 10) and (11) are very usefull in *in-vitro* tests. Using these Equations, one can analyse the mechanistic nature of drug release from the dosage form, by recording the amount of drug in the dissolution medium at each time point.

Usually, dissolution rate profiles appear to be linear (zero order), or exponential (first order), neither of which may actually represent the true mechanism and kinetics of drug release. It was recently demonstrated with microcapsules, under sink conditions, released their content by first order kinetics, actually released their drug at a zero order rate. It was the log normal distribution phenomena that caused the bulk release rate profile to appear as first order [95].

5.2 Pharmacokinetic Evaluation

It is expected that the pharmacokinetic profile of a well designed controlled release drug delivery system will differ from that of a conventional dosage from by minimizing blood levels spikes, and large osscilations in blood-drug levels.

Theoretical pharmacokinetic models describing the fate of a drug in the body, following oral administration of a controlled release dosage form, have been described in the literature as early as the 1960's and 1970's [96-98]. The most common approach in these models is to employ an initial, rapidly releasing drug fraction to quickly establish a blood drug level, together with a controlled release fraction to maintain the desired level. The controlled release fraction was modelled to release drug either by first-order or preferably, zero-order. This analysis, compartmental in nature, assumed that (1) first order kinetics governs the biological pathways of the drug, (2) drug absorption and elimination are irreversible, (3) complete absorption of the drug that has been released from the delivery system occurs, (4) release of drug from the dosage form is rate limiting. These assumptions are as valid today as they were twenty years ago, but the pharmacokinetic design has changed. A substantial number of controlled release drug delivery systems, that do not posses an immediate release fraction, were introduced to the pharmaceutical market. It thus became clear that the accumulation process is important to the therapeutic success of the products.

In the last decade, pharmacokinetic model-independent analysis became advantageous in relation to compartmental modelling. This type of analysis is based on statistical moment theory, in which the time course of drug concentration in biological fluids can be mathematically treated as a statistical distribution. Based on this theory, a mean residence time (MRT) is defined as the mean time that drug is involved in all kinetic processes, with no differentiation between absorption and disposition rate constants. The mathematical expression for MRT is as follows[99]:

$$MRT = \frac{\int_0^\infty tC\,dt}{\int_0^\infty C\,dt} = \frac{AUMC}{AUC} \quad (19)$$

where AUC is the area under the blood-drug concentration (C) versus time (t) curve and AUMC is the area under the product of concentration and time ($C \times t$) versus time (t) curve.

The MRT can serve as a tool to estimate quantitatively the degree of sustained release products, i.e., the more sustained the concentration in the biological fluids, the larger the MRT. By subtracting the value of MRT following intraveneous administration from the value of MRT after extravascular administration, the mean absorption time, MAT, is obtained:

$$MAT = MRT_{extravascular} - MRT_{intraveneous} \quad (20)$$

For first-order absorption: $MAT = 1/k_a$, and thus:

$$MRT_{oral} = MRT_{intraveneous} + 1/k_a \quad (21)$$

For zero-order absorption: $MAT = T/2$, and thus,

$$MRT_{oral} = MRT_{intraveneous} + T/2 \quad (22)$$

where T is the absorption time.

Equation 4, which describes the relationship between the therapeutic index (C_{max}/C_{min}), the elimination half life and the dosing interval (τ), can now be replaced by:

$$\tau \leqq 0.693\ MRT \frac{\ln C_{max}/C_{min}}{\ln 2} \quad (23)$$

The therapeutic index is important when discussing the relationship of delivery regimen, and the subsequent blood profile, to the safety and efficacy of the drug. Of no less importance is the dosage form index which may be defined as the ratio of maximum and minimum blood levels produced at steady state after multiple administration of a particular drug delivery system at a specific dosage regimen [100]. The dosage form index, or % fluctuations can be calculated according to the following Equation [101]:

$$\% \text{ fluctuations} = 100 \, \frac{\text{peak blood-concentration} - \text{trough blood-concentration}}{\text{trough blood-concentration}} \tag{24}$$

Most controlled release dosage forms are intended for chronic treatment, which means that multiple dose calculations must be considered in pharmacokinetic evaluations. Thus the peak and through blood-concentrations should be measured only after steady-state has been reached. The following Equations can be useful to calculate these parameters [24]:

$$C_{max(ss)} = \frac{D}{V} \cdot \frac{e^{-k_e t\,max}}{1 - e^{-k_e \tau}} \tag{25}$$

$$C_{min(ss)} = \frac{D}{V} \cdot \frac{k_a}{(k_a - k_e)} \left(\frac{e^{-k_e \tau}}{1 - e^{-k_e \tau}} - \frac{e^{-k_a \tau}}{1 - e^{-k_a \tau}} \right) \tag{26}$$

assuming complete absorption, where:

$$t_{max(ss)} = \frac{\ln \left[k_a(1 - e^{-k_e \tau})/k_e(1 - e^{-k_a \tau}) \right]}{k_a - k_e} \tag{27}$$

where D is the dose, V is the volume of distribution, k_e is the overall elimination rate constant, k_a is the absorption rate constant, and τ is the constant dosing interval.

5.3 Pharmacodynamic Evaluation

Halford and Sheiner have distinguished between "pharmacodynamic models" and "pharmacokinetic-Pharmacodynamic models" [102]. In the former the drug concentration can be determined at the site of action, whereas in the later, drug concentration is not measurable and the drug effect is used for quantitative kinetic analysis. They also defined pharmacodynamic models as those that are based on an equilibrium between drug concentration and drug effect. Since this equilibrium is not always achieved, a pharmacokinetic-pharmacodynamic model is required.

The linear model. The linear model is expressed by the following relationship:

$$E = S \cdot C + E_0 \tag{28}$$

where E is the therapeutic effect of the drug, E_0 is the effect measured without drug, C is the drug concentration and S is the slope of the linear curve obtained when plotting E versus C.

The log-linear model. When data cannot be fitted to the model represented by Eq. (28), a log-linear model is used:

$$E = S \cdot \log C + \text{Constant} \tag{29}$$

It should be emphasized that the data best fits such a model when the recorded effect is within the range of 20–80% of the maximum effect, given that an estimation of that maximum effect can be obtained.

The E_{max} and sigmoid E_{max} model. The E_{max} model takes into account the fact that the drug effect does not increase indefinitely as a function of drug concentration, but that it does have a maximum (E_{max}). The following hyperbolic Equation is typical of a saturable mechanism:

$$E = E_0 + \frac{E_{max} \cdot C}{C_{50} + C} \tag{30}$$

where E_{max} is the drug's maximum effect and C_{50} is the drug concentration producing 50% of E_{max}.

In certain circumstances a receptor site is capable of reacting with more than or less than one drug molecule. That is reflected by an exponent that is attached to C in Eq. (30), yielding a modified situation known as the sigmoid E_{max} model, represented by the following exponential Equation:

$$E = \frac{E_{max} \cdot C^n}{C_{50}^n + C^n} \tag{31}$$

Three typical curves of pharmacological response versus drug-blood level for different n values are shown in Fig. 8.

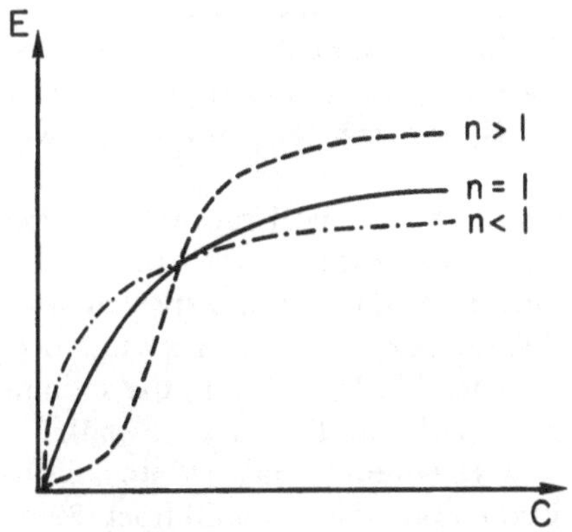

Fig. 8. Effect of the exponent n on the hyperbolic function of the E_{max} model for unsaturable relationship between pharmacologic effect and blood-drug concentration [102]

6 Issues in Controlled Drug Delivery

6.1 Population Differential and Clinical State

Pharmacokinetic and pharmacodynamic properties of controlled release dosage forms, are influenced by some additional factors that commonly are not taken into consideration at the development stage, e.g., population differential in metabolism, age or gender, disease states, and concomitant drug administration. Usually the blood level and pharmacological response following administration of new drug delivery systems, are studied in healthy volunteers, and conclusions are commonly made without satisfactory investigation of the clinical response of the patient. The pharmacodynamic response of children to some drugs is different from that of an adult [103]. Controlled release delivery systems are complicated in this instance as was previously demonstrated with theophylline sustained release products [104].

The geriatric population is an even more complex group because of its heterogenous nature: in many cases there is no correlation between the biological and chronological age and the rate of aging cannot be predicted [105]. Clinical reports indicate that the relation between pharmacokinetics and pharmacodynamics is different in this group. In many cases drug effects in the elderly do not correlate to the pharmacokinetic profiles found in younger populations. So is the case with physiological parameters influencing the performance of drug delivery systems like gastric emptying, which was reported to be longer in the elderly [106].

6.2 Physiological Considerations

As the number of publications and patents dealing with new drug delivery systems increase, it can be stated that sustained release technology is almost unlimited [107]. At the same time it can be stated that now, more than ever, the unknowns in this area are of great significance, such as the influence of the body physiology on the performance of drug delivery systems. Thus it is apparent that the biological response and pharmacokinetics of many drugs is subject to a circadian rhythm effect. Moreover, there are good reasons to expect that a constant supply of drug, i.e., zero order input to the receptor site, is unneccessary and that in many cases some other rate profile may be more appropriate. These types of perturbation can be built into the design of a controlled release drug delivery system. At present there does not appear to be any useful commercial examples of such systems but it is inevitable that these effects will be incorporated into future systems.

It is now clear that a lack of understanding of physiological processes during development of novel drug delivery systems, can yield inefficient control of drug release in the best cases, and tragedies in the worst cases. Thus, benoxaprofen after being approved by FDA, was found to be toxic due to unexpected drug accumulation and $t_{1/2}$ extension in elderly and renal failure patients [108]. In addition, the sodium indomethacin osmotic system has been reported to perforate the intestine wall [109].

Most controlled release drug delivery systems were developed taking into consideration normal motility or homogeneous absorption along the entire GI tract. Some systems did not consider Gl motility at all [110, 111, 79]. Furthermore, many drug delivery systems rely on manufacturing-control methods that do not reflect the real environment in which the drug is being released. Some manufacturers look at the Gl tract as a black box in which drug is being released and then absorbed in some way or another. This approach has already lead to undesired therapeutic phenomena such as dose dumping.

It is reasonable to state that, unlike research on new drugs, the research on drug delivery systems will concentrate in the next few years on a better understanding of biological and physiological processes important to drug delivery. This kind of research will enable scientists to optimize design and to make better use of existing controlled release dosage forms, as well as develop new and sophisticated drug carriers.

6.3 Future Trends

It is apparent that a major limitation of drug delivery is an inadequate understanding of drug disposition in the body at a fundamental level. This lack of understanding extends to patients and the variability associated with pathologies, age, gender, etc. It is this absence of a thorough understanding that limits our ability to optimize drug utilization through drug delivery.

One of the driving forces to extend our understanding of drug disposition is the fruits of advances in the biotechnology area, i.e., peptides/proteins. These sometimes large molecules, which are sensitive to enzymatic metabolism and immunologic processing, have significant constraints that limit their delivery. Attempts to understand and control these constraints will have a positive influence on the delivery of traditional drug molecules.

Thus, if the 1950's–1970's can be viewed as a period of technical approaches to controlled drug delivery, the 1980's and 1990's will be viewed as the biophysical period. Drug delivery will undoubtedly improve in sophistication as our knowledge base expands.

Table 7. Some Present and Projected Areas of Pharmaceutical Research

a. Continuous work in material sciences
b. Expanded activities in polymers:
   1. Improved biocompatibility;
   2. Better understanding and hence predictable of *in-vivo* performance
c. Expanded work in routes of drug delivery:
   1. Understanding of anatomy, physiology, biochemistry, and immunology;
   2. Better control of drug delivery through above subjects
d. Improvement in efficiency of processes
e. Expanded work on analogs and prodrugs
f. Expanded work on drug disposition within cells
g. Expanded work on solute interaction with cellular surface
h. Better understanding of pharmacodynamics and its relation to drug delivery systems
i. Stabilization and delivery of peptides and proteins
j. Improved and expanded interface at a good level between the physical-chemical-technology areas and the biological sciences

This review began with the comment that the drug delivery revolution was noisy without a great deal of commercial success. Despite the apparent lack of successful commercial products, there is significant continuous effort in an attempt to define what the problems are and in identification of a strategic plan and road map to address the many question-marks in controlled drug delivery.

Table 7 summarise some future trends in pharmaceutical research [112].

7 References

1. Prescott, L. F.: Historical review and perspective of rate control in drug therapy, in: Rate Control in Drug Therapy, (eds) Prescott, L. F., and Nimmo, W. S., p. 1, Edinburgh, Churchill Livingstone, 1985
2. Thompson, H. O., and Lee, C. O.: J. Amer. Pharm. Assoc. Sci. Ed. *34*, 135 (1945)
3. Banker, G. S.: Pharmaceutical application of controlled release: an overview of the past, present, and future, in: Medical Application of Controlled Release, Vol. II (eds) Langer, R. S., and Wise, D. L., p. 1, Boca Raton, C.R.C. Press, 1984
4. Chien, V. W., and Robinson, J. R.: Parent. Sci. Tech., *36* (6), 231 (1982)
5. Kadish, A. H.: Trans. Am. Soc. Artif. Intern. Organs., *9*, 363 (1963)
6. Irsigler, K., Kritz, H., and Lovett, R. G.: Controlled drug delivery in the treatment of diabetes mellitus, in: Critical Reviews in Therapeutic Drug Carrier Systems (ed) Bruck, S. D., C.R.C. Press, *1* (3), 189 (1985)
7. Schwartz, J. B.: Optimization techniques in pharmaceutical formulations and processing, in: Modern Pharmaceuticas (eds) Banker, G. S., and Rhodes, C. T., p. 711, New York, Marcel Dekker, 1979
8. Bohidar, N. R., Restaino, F. A., and Schwartz, J. B.: Drug Dev. Ind. Pharm. *5* (2) 175 (1979)
9. Gibaldi, M.: Biopharmaceutics and Clinical Pharmacokinetics, p. 113, Lea & Febiger, 1984
10. Theeuwes, F., and Bayne, W.: J. Pharm. Sci., *66* (10), 1388 (1977)
11. Levy, G.: Arch. Int. Pharmacodynam. Ther., *3*, 241 (1964)
12. Brockmeier, D., Voegele, D., von Hattingberg, H. M.: Arzneimittel-Forschung, *33*, 598 (1983)
13. Theeuwes, F.: In vitro validation of rate-controlled formulations and devices, in: Rate Control in Drug Therapy (eds) Prescott, L. F., and Nimmo, W. S., p. 121, Edinburgh, Churchill Livingstone, 1985
14. Stella, V. J., and Himmelstein, K. J.: Prodrugs: a chemical approach to targetted drug delivery, in: Directed Drug Delivery: A Multidisciplinary Approach (eds) Borchardt, R. T., Repta, A. R., and Stella, V. J., p. 247, Clifton, Humana Press, 1985
15. Juliano, R. L.: Microparticulate drug carriers: liposomes, microspheres and cells, in: Sustained and Controlled Release Drug Delivery Systems (eds) Robinson, J. R., and Lee, V. H., New York, Marcel Dekker Inc. 1987[2]
16. Poznansky, M. S., and Juliano, R. L.: Pharm. Rev., *36* (4), 277 (1984)
17. Poste, G., and Kirsh, R.: Biotechnology, *1*, 869
18. Kao, Y. J., and Juliano, R. L.: Biochem. Biophys. Acta., *677*, 453 (1981)
19. Hsu, M. J., and Juliano, R. L., ibid., *720*, 411 (1982)
20. Arturson, P., Laakso, T., and Edman, P.: J. Pharm. Sci., *72*, 1415 (1983)
21. Florence, A. T.: Rate controle in targetted drug delivery, in: Rate Control in Drug Therapy (eds) Prescott, L. F., and Nimmo, W. S., p. 103, Edinburgh, Curchill Livingstone, 1985
22. Conrad, J. M., and Robinson, J. R.: Sustained drug release from tablets and particles through coating, in: Pharmaceutical Dosage Forms: Tablets, Vol. 3, (eds) Lieberman, H. A., and Lachman, L., p. 149, New York, Marcel Dekker, 1982
23. Park, K., Wood, R., and Robinson, J. R.: Oral controlled release systems, in: Medical Applications of Controlled Release (eds) Langer, R. S., and Wise, D. L., Vol. 1, p. 159, Boca Raton, C.R.C. Press, 1984
24. Gibaldi, M., and Perrier, D.: Pharmacokinetics, p. 188. New York, Marcel Dekker, 1982[2]

25. Ritschel, W. A.: Handbook of Basic Pharmacokinetics, p. 345, Hamilton, Drug Intelligence Publications, 1980[2]
26. Lee, V. H., and Robinson, J. R.: Methods to achieve sustained drug delivery, in: sustained and Controlled Release Drug Delivery Systems, (ed) Robinson, J. R., p. 123, New York, Marcel Dekker, 1978
27. Hixon, A. W., and Crowell, J. H.: Ind. Eng. Chem., *23*, 923 (1931)
28. Patel, M., and Carstensen, J. T.: J. Pharm. Sci., *64*, 1651 (1975)
29. Heller, J., and Trescony, P. V.: J. Pharm. Sci., *68*, 919 (1979)
30. Flynn, G. L.. Yalkowsky, S. H., and Roseman, T. J.: J. Pharm. Sci. *63* (4), 479 (1974)
31. Higuchi, T.: J. Pharm. Sci., *52*, 1145 (1963)
32. Benita, S.: Labo. Pharma-Probl. Tech., *32* (346), 694 (1984)
33. Theeuwes, F.: J. Pharm. Sci., *64*, 1987 (1975)
34. Schacht, E. H.: Ionic polymers as drug carriers, in: Controlled Drug Delivery, Vol. 1, Basic Concepts, (ed) Bruck, S. D., p. 149, Florida, C.R.C. Press, 1983
35. Raghunathan, Y., Amsel, L., Hinsvack, O., and Bryant, W.: J. Pharm. Sci. *70*, 379 (1981)
36. Brodin, A. E., Kavaliunas, D. R., and Frank, S. G.: Acta Pharm. Suecia. *15* (1), 1 (1978)
37. Nash, R. A.: Drug Cosmetic Ind. *97*, 843 (1965)
38. Collard, R. E.: Pharm. J. *186*, 113 (1962)
39. Gray, J. E.: Pathological evaluation of injection injury, in: Sustained and Controlled Release Drug Delivery Systems, (ed) Robinson, J. R., p. 351, New York, Marcel Dekker, 1978
40. Thompson, R. E., and Hecht, R. A.: Amer. J. Clin. Nutr. *7*, 311 (1959)
41. Chien, Y. W.: J. Parent. Sci. Tech. *35*, 106 (1981)
42. Salama, G., Hautecouverture, N., and Assan, R.: Diabetes *23*, 732 (1974)
43. Sefton, M. V.: Implantable pumps, in: Medical applications of Controlled Release (eds) Langer, R. S., and Wise, D. L., Vol. 1; p. 129, Florida, C.R.C. Press, 1984
44. Marliss, E. B., Caron, D., Albisser, A. M., and Zinman, B.: Diabetes Care *4*, 325 (1981)
45. Bolick, T., and Walker, M.: Diabetes, *30* (Suppl. 1) (Abstr.), 265 (1981)
46. Buchwald, H., Grage, T. B., Vassilopoulos, P. P., Rohde, T. D., Varco, R. L., and Blackshear, P.: Cancer *45*, 886 (1980)
47. Mckinstry, D. W.: Res. Resources Rep. *5*, 1 (1981)
48. Buchwald, H., Rohde, T. D., Schneider, P. D., Varco, R. L., and Blackshear, P. J.: Surgery *88*, 507 (1980)
49. Langer, R.: Pharmac. Ther., *21*, 35 (1983)
50. Blackshear, P. J., Dorman, F. D., Blackshear, P. L., Varco, R. L., and Buchwald, H.: Surg. Gynec. Obstet., *134*, 51 (1972)
51. Notari, R. E.: Pharmac. Ther. *14*, 25 (1981)
52. Sinkula, A. A.: Methods to achieve sustained drug delivery: the chemical approach, in: Sustained and Controlled Release Drug Delivery Systems (ed). Robinson, J. R., p. 411, New York, Marcell Dekker, (1978)
53. Julou, L., Bourat, G., Ducrot, R., Foumrel, J., and Garret, C.: Acta Psychiat. Scand. *49*, Suppl, 241, 9 (1973)
54. Loiseau, P., Brachet, A., and Hery, P.: Epilepsia *16*, 609 (1975)
55. Bialer, M., Rubinstein, A., Dubrowsky, J., Raz, I., and Abramsky, O.: Int. J. Pharm., *23*, 25 (1985)
56. Rubinstein, A., Bialer, M., Friedman, M., Raz, I., and Abramsky, O.: J. Controlled Release, 4, 33, 1986
57. Bodor, N.: Med. Res. Rev. *4* (4), 449 (1984)
58. Poznansky, M. J., and Cleland, L. G.: Biological macromolecules as carriers of drugs and enzymes, in: Drug Delivery Systems, Characteristics and Biomedical Applications, (ed) Juliano, R. L., p. 253, New York, Oxford University Press, 1980
59. Levin, V. A., Patlak, C. S., and Landahl, H. D.: J. Pharmacokin. Biopharm. *8*, 257 (1980)
60. Levin, V. A., Landahl, H. D., and Patlak, C. S.: Cancer Treat. Rep. *65 Suppl 2*, 19 (1981)
61. Bangham, A. D.: Ann. Rev. Biochem. *41*, 753 (1972)
62. Juliano, R. L.: Interaction of proteins and drugs with liposomes, in: Liposomes, (ed) Ostro, M., pp. 53, New York, Marcel Dekker, 1984
63. Poste, G., Kirsh, R., Fogler, W. E., and Fidler, I. J.: Cancer Res. *39*, 881 (1979)

64. Fidler, I. J.: Science *208* (4451), 1469 (1980)
65. Deodhar, S. D., James, K., Chiang, T., Edinger, M., and Barna, B. P.: Cancer Res. *41* (12), 5084 (1982)
66. Deodhar, S. D., Gautam, S., Yen Liberman, B., and Roberts, D.: Cancer Res. *44* (1), 305 (1984)
67. Herman, E. H., Rahman, A., Ferrans, V. J., Vick, J. A., and Schein, P. S.: Cancer Res. *43* (11), 5427 (1983)
68. Mehta, R., Lopez-Berestein, G., Hopfer, R., Mills, K., and Juliano, R. L.: Biochem. Biophys. Acta *770* (2), 230 (1984)
69. New, R. R. C., Chance, M. L., Thomas, S. C., and Peters, W.: Nature *272*, 55 (1978)
70. Zimmerman, U., Pilwat, G., and Esser, B.: J. Clin. Chem. Clin. Biochem., *16*, 135 (1978)
71. Ihaler, G. M.: Pharmac. Ther. *20*, 151 (1983)
72. Yelton, D. E., and Scharff, M. D.: Ann. Rev. Biochem. *50*, 657 (1981)
73. Neville, D. M.: Monoclonal antibody mediated drug delivery and antibody toxin conjugates, in: Directed Drug Delivery a Multidiciplinary Approach, p. 211, (eds) Borchardt, R. T., Repta, A. J., and Stella, V. J. Clifton, Humana Press, 1985
74. Gregoriadis, G.: Drugs *24*, 261 (1982)
75. Morimoto, Y., Okumura, M., Sugibayashi, K., and Kato, Y.: J. Pharm. Dyn. *4*, 624 (1981)
76. Hsieh, D. S., Langer, R., and Folkman, J.: Proc. Natl. Acad. Sci. U.S.A. *78* (3), 1863 (1981)
77. Robinson, J. R.: Recent advances in topical drug delivery, in: Rate Control in Drug Therapy (eds) Prescott, L. F., and Nimmo, W. S., p. 71, Edinburgh, Churchill Livingstone, 1985
78. Davis, S. S., Hardy, J. G., Taylor, M. J., Whalley, D. R., and Wilson, C. G.: Int. J. Pharm. *21*, 167 (1984)
79. Meyer, J. H., Dressman, J., Fink, A., and Amidon, G.: Gastroenterology *89*, 805 (1985)
80. Bechgaard, H., and Ladefoged, K.: J. Pharm. Pharmac. *30*, 690 (1978)
81. Park, K., and Robinson, J. R.: Int. J. Pharm. *19*, 107 (1984)
82. Park, H., and Robinson, J. R.: J. Contr. Rel. *2*, 47 (1985)
83. Machida, Y., Masuda, H., Fujiyama, N., Ito, S., Iwata, M., and Nagai, T.: Chem. Pharm. Bull. *27* (1), 93 (1979)
84. Machida, Y., Masuda, H., Fujiyama, N., Iwata, M., and Nagai, T.: Chem. Pharm. Bull *28* (4), 1125 (1980)
85. Gurney, R., Meyer, J. M., and Peppas, N. A.: Biomaterials *5*, 336 (1984)
86. Longer, M. A., Ch'ng, H. S., and Robinson, J. R.: J. Pharm. Sci. *74* (4), 406 (1985)
87. Welling, P. G.: Pharm. Int. *1*, 14 (1980)
88. Smart, J. D., Kellaway, I. W., and Worthington, E. C.: J. Pharm. Pharmacol. *36*, 295 (1984)
89. Gibaldi, M. H.: Pros. Clin. Pharmacol. *3* (2), 9 (1985)
90. Guy, R. H., and Hadgraft, J.: J. Pharm. Int. *112*, May (1985)
91. Gibaldi, M. H.: ibid. *3* (3), 17 (1985)
92. The United States Pharmacopeia, Twenty First Revision, United States Pharmacopeial Convention Inc., p. 1243, Rockville, 1985
93. Simmons, D. L., Frechette, M., Ranz, R. J., Chen, N. S., and Patel, N. K.: Can. J. Pharm. Sci. 7; 62 (1972)
94. Peppas, N. A.: Mathematical models for controlled release kinetics, in: Medical Applications of Controlled Release, Vol. II (ed) Langer, R. S., and Wise, D. L., p. 169, Florida, C.R.C. Inc., 1984
95. Hoffmann, A., Donbrow, M., Gross, S. T., and Benita, S.: Correlation of individual and Global release profiles from microcapsules, in: Proceedings of the 12th International Symposium on Controlled Release of Bioactive Materials, July 1985, (eds) Peppas, N. A., and Haluska, R., J. Lincolnshire, Controlled Release Soc., 1985
96. Rowland, M., and Beckett, A. H.: J. Pharm. Pharmacol. *16S*, 156T (1964)
97. Robinson, J. R., and Eriksen, S.P.: J. Pharm. Sci. *55*, 1254 (1966)
98. Dobrinska, M. R., and Welling, P. G.: J. Pharm. Sci. *64*, 1728 (1975)
99. Riegelman, S., and Collier, P.: J. Pharmacokin. Biopharm. *8*, 509 (1980)
100. Heimlich, K. R.: Curr. Med. Res. Op. *8*, *Suppl. 2*, 28 (1983)
101. Gibaldi, M. H.: Clin. Pharmacol. *2*, 25 (1984)
102. Halford, N. H. G., and Scheiner, L. B.: Pharmac. Ther. *66*, 143 (1982)
103. Green, T. P., and Mirkin, B. L.: Clinical pharmacokinetics: pediatric considerations, in: Phar-

macokinetic Basis for Drug Treatment, (eds) Benet, L. Z., Massound, N., and Gambertoglio, J. G., p. 269, New York, Raven Press, 1984
104. NIH Theophylline Workshop, September 4–6, 1985, Bethesda, MD
105. Ferraiolo, B. L., and Benet, L. Z.: Pharmacodynamic considerations in the development of new drug delivery concepts, in: Directed Drug Delivery (eds) Borchardt, R. T., Repta, A. J., and Stella, V. J., p. 13, New Jersey, Humana Press, 1985
106. Evans, M. A., Triggs, E. J., Cheung, M., Broe, G. A., and Creasey, H.: J. Am. Ger. Soc. *XXIX* (5), 201 (1981)
107. Check, W. A.: Amer. J. Hosp. Pharm. *41*, 1536 (1984)
108. Roth, S. H.: Arch. Intern. Med. *144*, 472 (1984)
109. Adverse Reactions, in: The Pharmaceutical Journal p. 203, Aug. 20, 1983
110. Barr, W. H.: Pharmacotherapy *4(4)*, 167 (1984)
111. Nimmo, W. S.: Pharm. Int. 221 Nov. (1980)
112. Robinson, J. R.: Pharmaceutics and the evolving technology of drug delivery — a perspective, in: Directed Drug Delivery (eds) Borchardt, R. T., Repta, A. J., and Stella, V. J., p. 3, New Jersey, Humana Press, 1985

Enzyme-Immunoassay: A Review

A. Hubbuch, E. Debus, R. Linke, and W. J. Schrenk

Boehringer Mannheim Gmbh, Sandhofer Straße 116, 6800 Mannheim, BRD

The rapid expansion of immunoassays is due to their remarkable specificity and sensitivity, allowing the quantitation of a large variety of structures. In the last few years enzyme-immunoassays in particular have found wide acceptance in clinical laboratories.

The aim of this review is to present the versatility of enzyme-immunoassays with respect to their broad spectrum of methods and analytes. Special attention has been given to the performance characteristics of enzyme-immunoassays and to some antibody reagents used in separation enzyme-immunoassays.

1 Introduction

Enzyme-immunoassays (EIAs) have come a long way in a relatively short time. While not much more than a decade ago, clinical and laboratory physicians had asked themselves whether the obvious handling advantages compared to radio-immunoassays could outweigh the drawbacks such as lack of sensitivity and moderate precision, today's EIAs measure low molecular weight haptens such as T_3, fT_4, or digoxin just as sensitively and reliably as any isotope method [1-7]; the same holds true for high molecular weight proteins in very low serum concentrations such as CEA, hCG, TSH and many others.

Many reviews (e.g. [5-7, 12-14]), several monographs (e.g. [15-29]) and practical guides to set up EIAs (e.g. [30-35]) have already been published. As it is almost impossible to discuss all aspects of EIA in one review article, this paper will concentrate on the most important principles, applications and performance characteristics as well as some antibody reagents.

It started in 1971 when two groups [8, 9] described a new type of immunoassay, using an enzymic instead of a radioactive label: the enzyme-linked immunosorbent assay (ELISA). Analogous to the classical radioimmunoassay (RIA) of Yalow and Berson [10], this technique involves a separation of the solid phase-bound antigen-antibody complex from the unbound (= free) fraction ("bound/free separation"). Already one year later, Rubinstein described another EIA not requiring a bound/free separation [11]. Based on these two principle techniques, EIAs can be subdivided into two groups, commonly named heterogeneous and homogeneous EIAs. Since not all EIAs termed homogeneous really are homogeneous assays, the more descriptive and more accurate terms separation (or separation required) and non-separation (or separation-free) should be used [25].

In separation methods an antibody or antigen is bound to a solid phase and a bound/free separation is necessary. In non-separation methods the antigen/antibody interaction modifies the activity of the enzyme, which allows a quantitative evaluation in homogeneous phase.

Among the non-isotopic immunoassays available today [36-42] EIA in particular has proved to be an especially suitable alternative to RIA. Enzymes, coenzymes and enzyme-inhibitors are commonly used as markers [7], which allow an easy detection by instruments routinely used in the measurement of enzyme activities.

2 Types of Enzyme-Immunoassays

2.1 *Non-separation Enzyme-Immunoassay*

The development of most non-separation enzyme-immunoassays follows a similar pattern. In brief the recipe reads:

1. Choose an appropriate enzyme/substrate system.
2. Couple hapten and/or antibody (fragment) with:

— an enzyme, e.g. EMIT® [5,11,19], THERESIA [43,44];
— a substrate or substrate precursor, e.g. SLFIA [45];
— an enzyme inhibitor, e.g. EMMIA [46–49];
— a prosthetic group, e.g. ARIS [50–53];
— a liposome containing an enzyme [54,55];
— a cytotoxic agent for liposomes with entrapped enzyme [56];
— a pair of cooperating enzymes, e.g. channelling EIA [57) 58].

3. Modulate the enzyme-substrate reaction by means of the antigen/antibody reaction: increasing amounts of hapten within the reaction mixture increases or decreases the substrate turnover, which is detected photometrically.

The basic idea for non-separation enzyme immunoassays was the discovery that some antibodies against enzymes can inhibit the catalytic activity by formation of the antibody-enzyme complex [59,60], see Fig. 1. This principle is applied to the convenient measurement of diagnostically relevant enzymes, notable iso-enzymes such as creatine kinase MB subunits [60,157], see also page 115. A similar behaviour is observed if appropriate hapten-enzyme conjugates are used [11]. As a fairly high number of non-separation enzyme-immunoassays has been developed in the recent years [5,17–31], only some examples can be mentioned within this review.

The EMIT® (Syva-Merck GmbH, Darmstadt, FRG) takes advantage of this hapten-induced modulation and is the most widely used homogeneous system (Fig. 2). Several explanations are possible for the inhibition of the haptenized enzyme bound to the antibody: steric hindrance, conformational change of the enzyme, or prevention of a conformational change necessary for enzyme activity. An exception to this mechanism is the thyroxine assay, where antibody activates the antibody-bound enzyme-hapten conjugate [5].

Another non-separation EIA is represented by ARIS (apoenzyme-reactivation-immunoassay, Fig. 3): In this method a hapten such as theophylline is coupled to FAD [50]. The antibody against theophylline inhibits FAD to form an active enzyme complex with the glucose-oxidase apoenzyme. Free theophylline competes with the

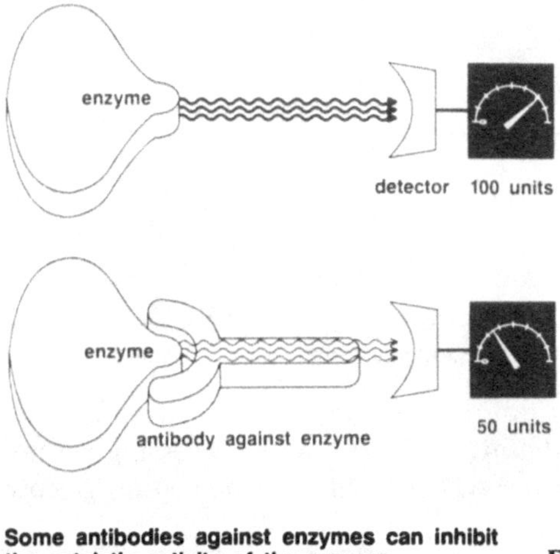

Fig. 1. Experimental basis for non-separation EIAs

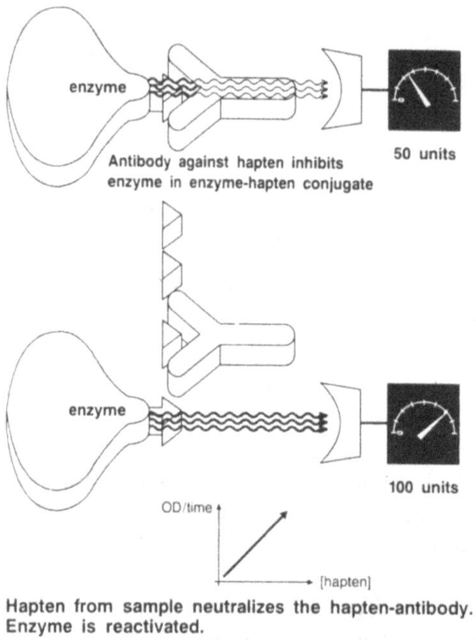

Fig. 2. Experimental basis for EMIT®

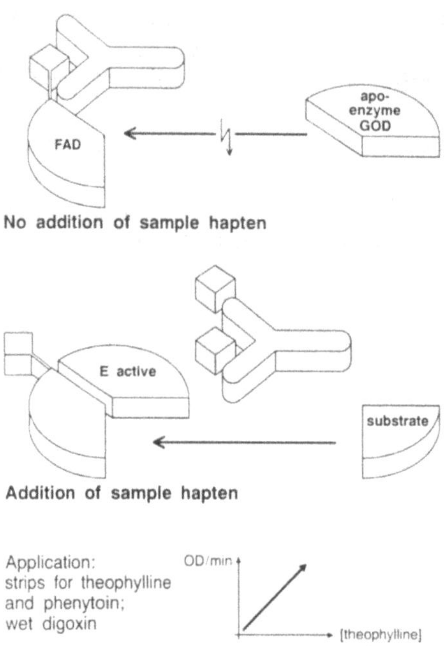

Fig. 3. Non-separation EIA of type ARIS (apoenzyme-reactivation-immuno-assay)

theophylline-FAD conjugate for the inhibiting antibody. With increasing serum-theophylline concentration more haptenized FAD is freed, thus activating glucose oxidase.

In the substrate-labelled fluorescence-immunoassay (SLFIA) hapten is coupled

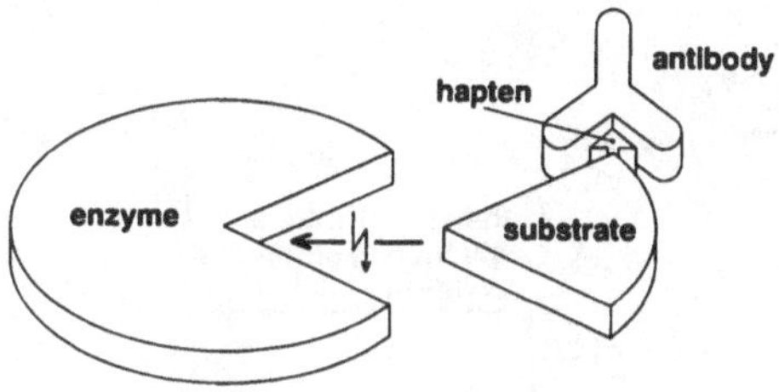

Fig. 4. Substrate labelled enzyme-immunoassay (SLFIA)

with the fluorigenic substrate of the enzyme β-galactosidase (Fig. 4). If the labelled hapten is bound to the antibody, the β-galactosidase activity is inhibited: enzyme activity increases with increasing hapten concentrations [45].

In the inhibitor-labelled EIA hapten is bound to an inhibitor of the enzyme (Fig. 5). With increasing hapten concentrations the inhibitor is freed from the antibody-hapten complex, which leads to an inhibition of the enzyme: the enzyme activity is inversely proportional to the hapten concentration in the sample [46-49]:

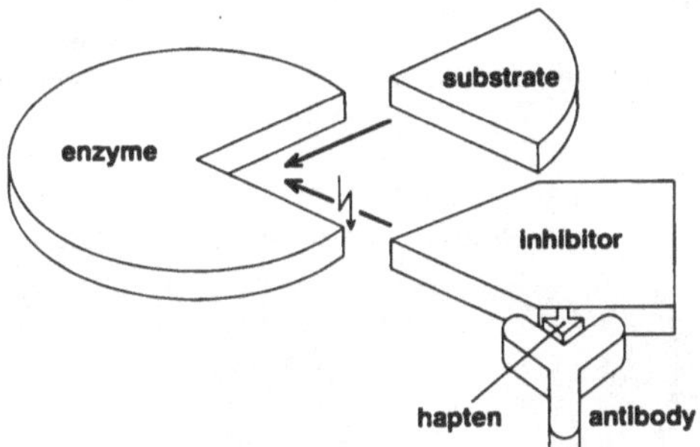

Fig. 5. Inhibitor labelled enzyme-immunoassay

The enzyme-channeling EIA is based on the observation that the initial rate of product (P_2) formation of two consecutive enzyme-catalysed reactions is increased, if the two enzymes are brought close together (e.g. by co-immobilization on the same solid support or by means of an appropriate antigen-antibody complex) [57,58,61]. Usually a scavenger enzyme (E_3) is added in order to minimize background reaction caused by uncomplexed/free enzymes E_1 and E_2.

$$S \xrightarrow{E_1} \underset{\substack{\downarrow \\ Q}}{P_1} \underset{E_3}{\xrightarrow{E_2}} P_2$$

Figure 6 shows the application on a test-strip procedure utilizing a combination of immuno-capillary migration and enzyme-channelling. The height of the colour front on the strip is proportional to the analyte concentration, e.g. theophylline [62].

A quite different approach is taking advantage of liposome-entrapped enzymes. One popular modification of this EMIA (enzyme-membrane-immunoassay, Fig. 7) is the use of haptenized liposomes [54,55].

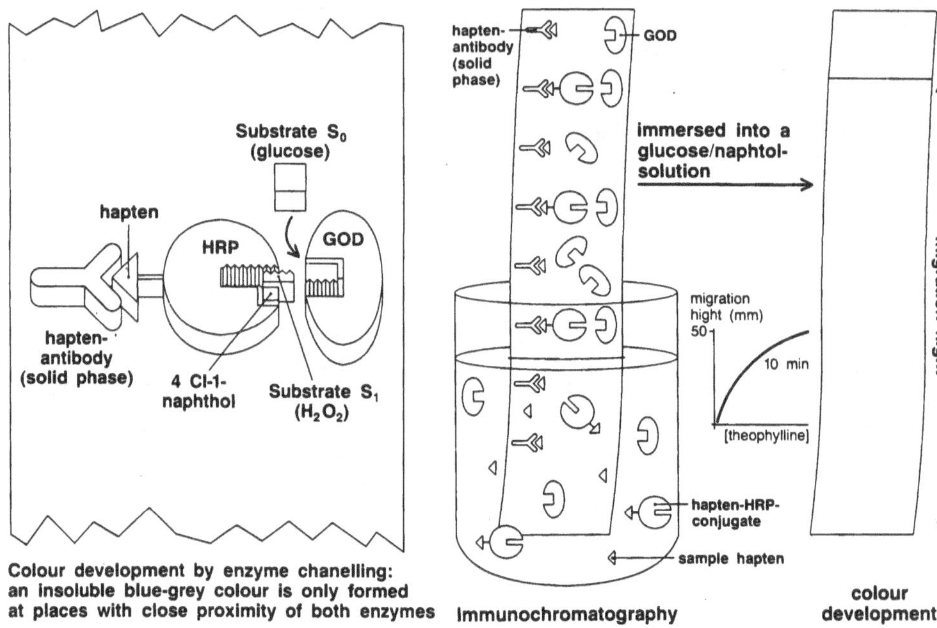

a b

Fig. 6. Enzyme-chanelling immunoassay; principle (**a**) and application in a test strip procedure (**b**)

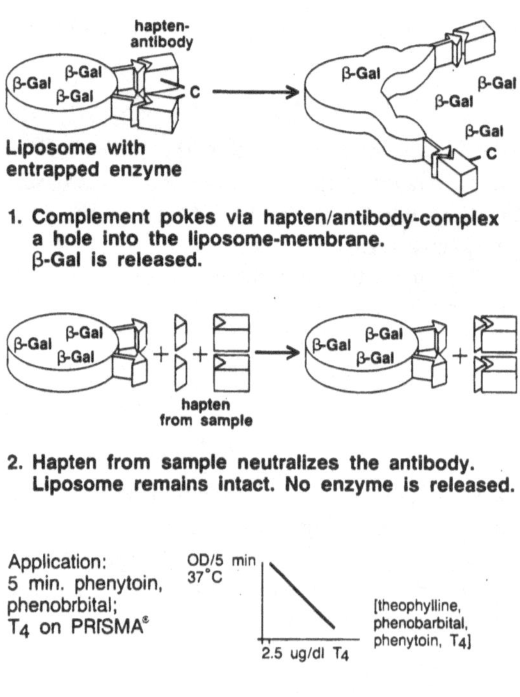

Fig. 7. Non-separation EIA of type EMIA (enzyme-membrane-immunoassay) with haptenized liposomes

Via the antigen/antibody reaction, complement pokes a hole into the membrane of β-galactosidase-filled liposomes. Entrapped β-galactosidase is released and can be measured as usual. Addition of hapten-containing serum neutralizes the antibody. The liposomes remain intact, no enzyme is released, thus no enzyme activity can be measured.

In a modification of the above principle cytolysine is used instead of complement [56], Fig. 8: alkaline phosphatase is entrapped in the liposome. As long as the haptenized cytolysine is bound to the antibody, the membrane is not affected. The hapten-cytolysine conjugate is liberated after addition of a hapten-containing serum sample, which is followed by lysis of the membrane and release of alkaline phosphatase: hapten "activates" the enzyme.

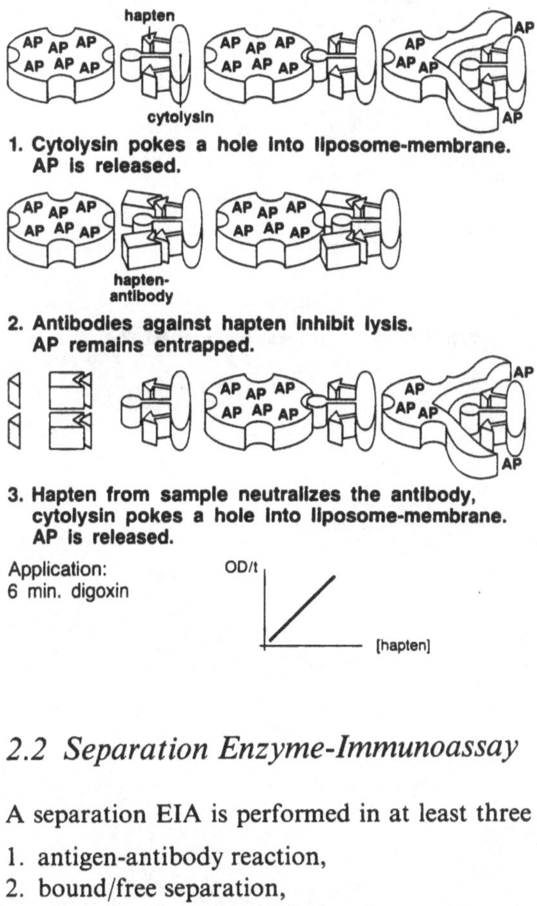

Fig. 8. Non-separation EIA of EMIA-type (enzyme-membrane-immunoassay) with haptenized cytolysin

2.2 *Separation Enzyme-Immunoassay*

A separation EIA is performed in at least three steps:

1. antigen-antibody reaction,
2. bound/free separation,
3. enzyme-substrate reaction and spectrometric measurement.

A large variety of techniques utilizing this principle has been developed during the recent years [15-29].

Iso-enzymes, such as prostatic acid phosphatase [158-160] and pancreatic α-amylase [161] can easily by determined following the specific reaction with an antibody. In case of pancreatic α-amylase, for instance, human salivary amylase is bound to a monoclonal antibody and inhibited. The remaining pancreatic amylase activity is measured with a routine method [161].

The competitive enzyme-immunoassay is very similar to the well-known classical radioimmunoassay of Yalow and Berson [62]. It involves competition between labelled and unlabelled antigen for a limited amount of antigen-specific antibody (Fig. 9). The amount of solid-phase-bound enzyme-labelled antigen can be measured photometrically and is inversely proportional to the concentration of unlabelled antigen present [5,63].

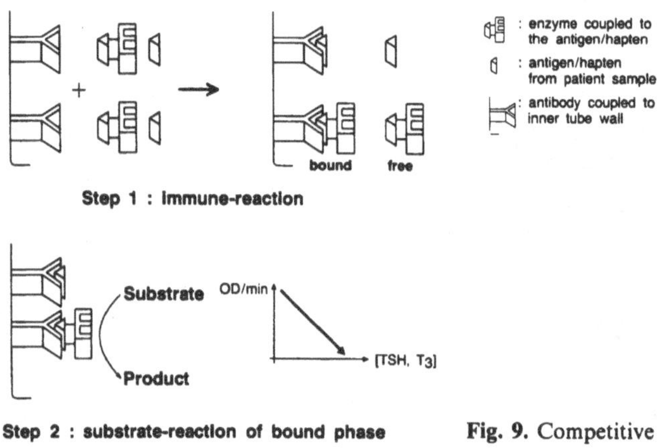

Fig. 9. Competitive test mode of separation EIA

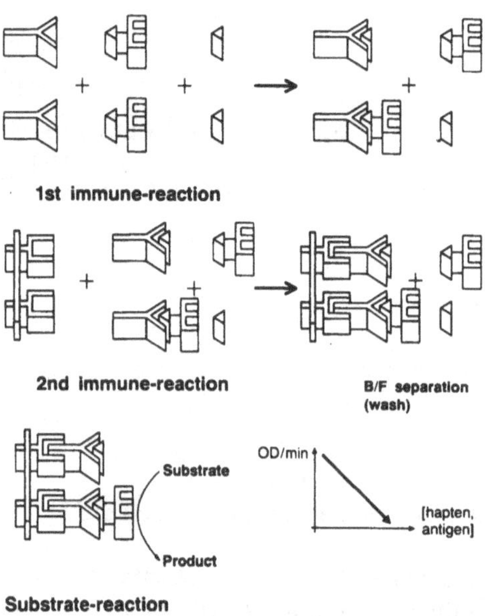

Fig. 10. DALP (double antibody liquid phase), a rapid separation EIA

A faster reacting type of competitive tests is represented by the DALP (double-antibody liquid phase) technique [64], Fig. 10). Differing from the reaction sequence shown in Fig. 9, the (first) antigen-antibody reaction takes place in homogeneous phase. In the second step all antigen-antibody complexes are bound to a second solid phase-bound antibody. The subsequent bound/free separation gets rid of all serum material and the enzyme-substrate reaction proceeds as usual.

Whereas competitive tests are working with enzyme-labelled antigens, the immuno-enzymometric method (IEMA, Fig. 11) utilizes enzyme-labelled antibodies and solid phase-bound antigens [65,66].

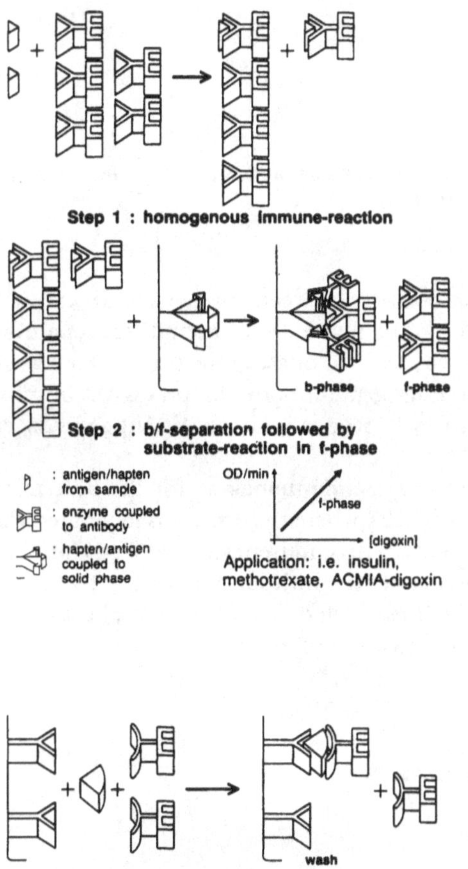

Fig. 11. Immune-enzymometric-assay (IEMA)

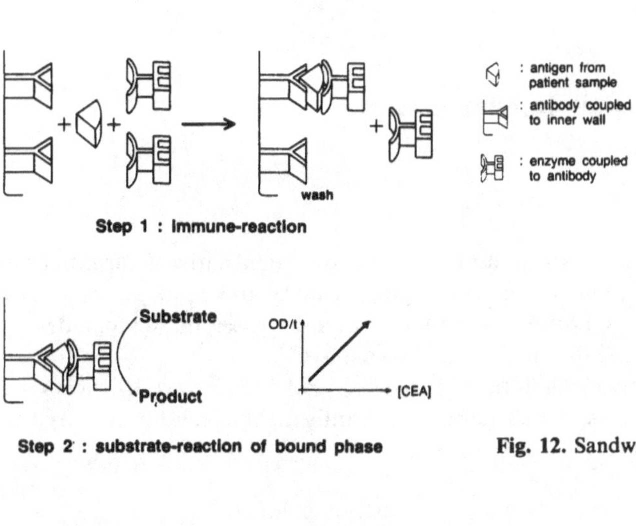

Fig. 12. Sandwich-test-mode

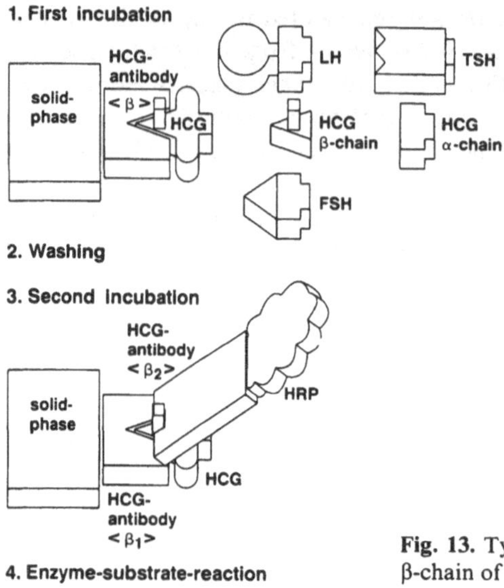

Fig. 13. Typical two-step-sandwich-EIA for hCG (and free β-chain of hCG)

As with the DALP-technique, the first reaction between antigen and an excess of enzyme-labelled antibody takes place in the liquid phase. In the bound/free separation step the excess of labelled antibody is removed by solid phase antigen and after a washing step the enzymatic activity of the soluble antigen/antibody complexes can be measured photometrically. The enzymatic activity is proportional to the antigen concentration.

The most widely distributed separation enzyme-immunoassay for the determination of proteins is the sandwich test [19,67], Fig. 12), where the protein is incubated with a large excess of solid phase-bound antibody. A second enzyme-labelled antibody, recognizing a different epitope of the protein antigen (without interference by the first antibody) is bound to the protein as well (Fig. 12 and 13). The solid phase-bound enzyme activity is proportional to the concentration of antigen.

3 Application of Enzyme-Immunoassays

3.1 Analytes

In principle, enzyme-immunoassays can be used for the quantitative determination of every compound to which antibodies with high specificity and avidity can be raised, such as antigens, antibodies, hormones, proteins, toxins, viruses and insecticides [6,30]. A very recent application is the field of DNA-analysis [68].

Extensive lists of analytes have been published [1,5,12,13]. Figure 14 shows some examples of diagnostically important haptens and antigens that can be measured with enzyme-immunoassays.

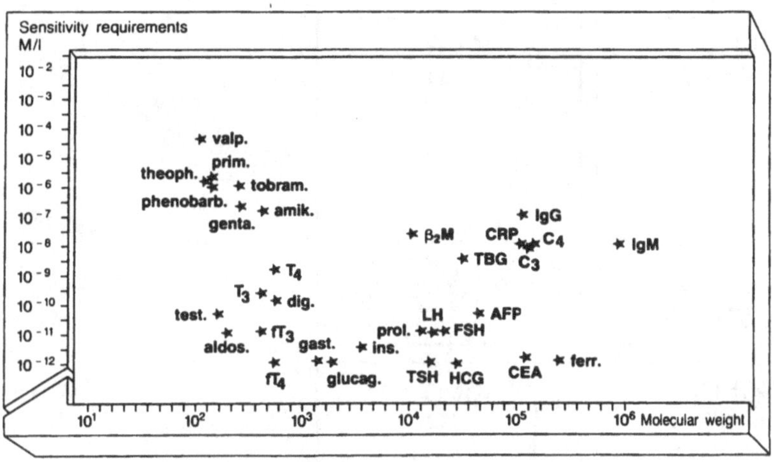

Fig. 14. Hormones, proteins and drugs of clinical interest

The majority of homogeneous enzyme-immunoassay-techniques is devoted to the routine measurement of small molecular weight haptens above serum concentrations of 10^{-9} mol/l. Typically drugs fall into that category. Few attempts were made to utilize non-separation enzyme-immunoassays for the measurement of proteins in serum concentrations above 10^{-9} mol/l, i.e. IgG [57,69,70] or CRP [71]. Practically all attempts failed to provide the routine laboratories with homogeneous EIAs that allow an easy determination of proteins being present in serum below 10^{-9} mol/l. In contrast, all the haptens and antigens having molecular weights from 500 Dalton to above 10^6 Dalton and being present in serum in concentrations from 10^{-3} mol/l to 10^{-12} mol/l (e.g. theophylline, T_3, TSH) are accessible to heterogeneous enzyme-immunoassay techniques (see Fig. 14).

3.2 Precision

In 1980 Oellerich [72] reported between-day coefficients of variation from 2 to 10% in the medium measuring range (duplicate determinations with partially or fully mechanized analysers). These data were rated to be of the same quality as those of corresponding radioimmunoassays.

Although in general these figures still are valid today, some improvements were achieved during the last five years. Three examples may demonstrate typical improvements:

- Normal and decreased serum TSH concentrations can be measured with low imprecision and the precision profiles in Fig. 15 show that a sandwich EIA (Enzymun-Test® TSH-S) may even be superior to some sandwich RIAs [3].
- With a fully mechanized analyzer (ES 600) for separation enzyme-immunoassays, the majority of CVs was found to be below 5% [73], Table 1. This is mainly due to the fact that such a system performs tests under rigidly controlled conditions of temperature and incubation time.

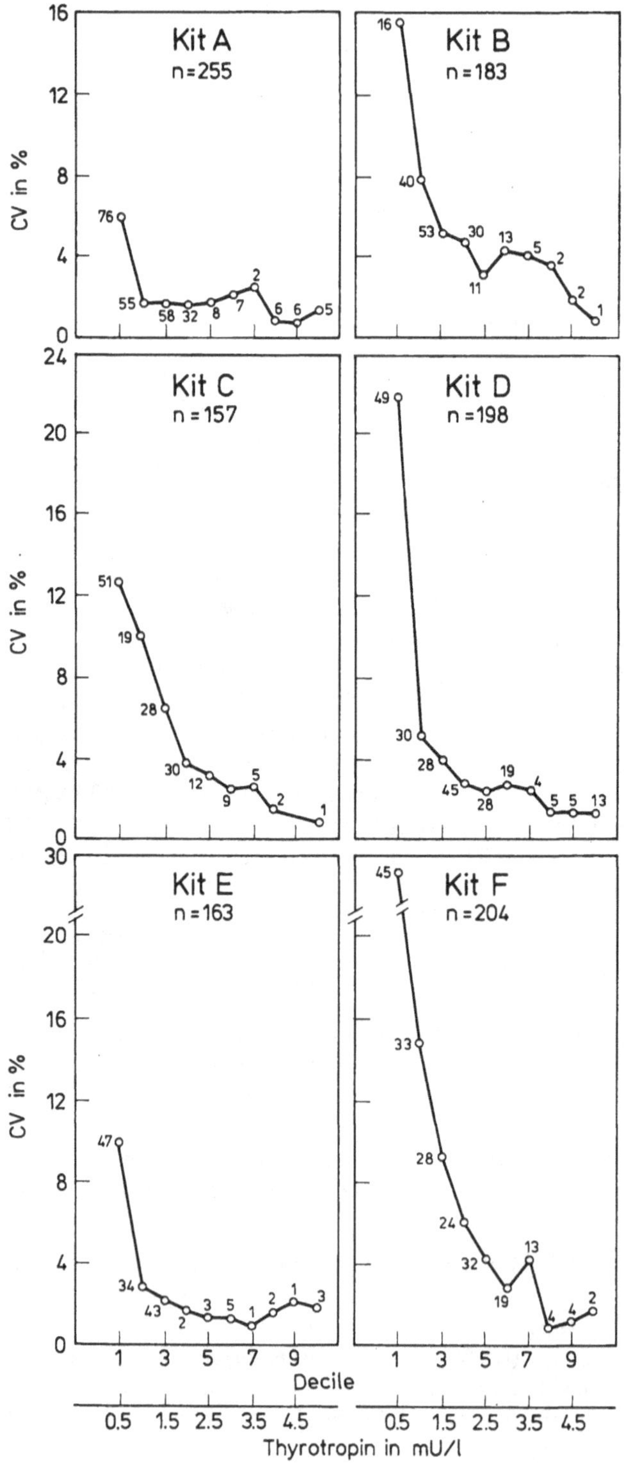
Kit A
n = 255
Kit B
n = 183
Kit C
n = 157
Kit D
n = 198
Kit E
n = 163
Kit F
n = 204
CV in %
Decile
Thyrotropin in mU/l

Table 1. Precision of Enzymun-Test® diagnostics on the fully mechanized analyzer ES 600. From: Willnow, P., Raichle, T., Scientific Bavaria 1985

test	unit	within series			day-to-day		
		x̄	SD	CV (%)	x̄	SD	CV (%)
T_3	ng/ml	1.88	0.06	3.2	2.90	0.07	2.4
T_4	µg/dl	19.1	0.40	2.1	8.60	0.96	11.1
TBG	ng/ml	18.8	0.62	3.3	18.9	1.42	7.5
DIGOXIN	ng/ml	1.38	0.02	1.4	1.38	0.05	3.7
DIGITOXIN	ng/ml	33.9	1.20	3.5	30.1	1.57	5.2
TSH	µU/ml	7.95	0.17	2.1	18.0	0.34	1.9
AFP	IU/ml	66.4	0.76	1.1	56.9	1.80	3.2
FERRITIN	ng/ml	196.8	5.11	2.6	221.0	4.09	1.9
CEA	ng/ml	20.6	0.25	1.2	27.7	0.71	2.6

— Figure 16 shows the improvement of precision with a partly mechanized analyzer compared to the manual procedure [74].

In many cases duplicate or triplicate determinations are no longer necessary because adequate precision can be achieved with single determinations.

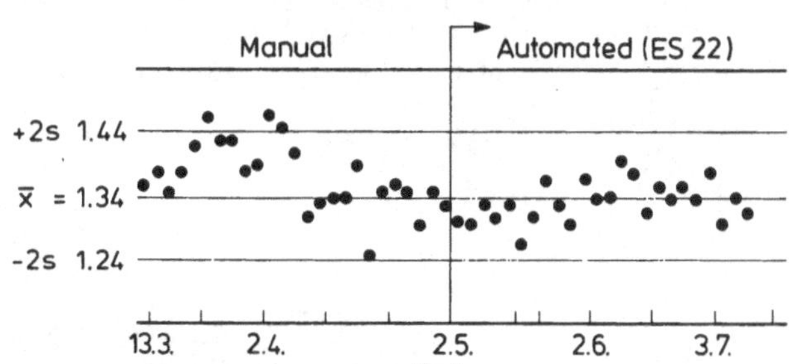

Fig. 16. Quality control chart for Enzymun-Test® TBK with manual and mechanized (ES 22) performance. From: Meyer, H. D., Braun, S. C.: Ärztl. Lab. *31*, 308 (1985)

◀

Fig. 15. The diagrammes show the compound precision profiles from 10 assays with each kit, using the values lying between the lower detection limit of the assay and 5 mU/l thyrotropin. The deciles represent concentration steps of 0.5 mU/l and the numbers by each point the number of data (from duplicate determinations) used in each decile. The total number of duplicates used is also shown for each kit.
Kit B: RIA (competition principle); Kit E: Sandwich EIA (Enzymun-Test® TSH S); Kits A, C, D, F: Sandwich RIA; From: Wood, W. G. et al., J. Clin. Chem. Clin. Biochem. *23*, 461 (1985)

3.3 Sensitivity and detection limits

Many of the early enzyme-immunoassays were less sensitive and had higher detection limits than comparable radioimmunoassays. This situation has changed and heterogeneous enzyme-immunoassays show detection limits and sensitivities that are comparable to those of radioimmunoassays. Detection limits are in the range of 10^{-12} mol/l 1 [75], see Fig. 14.

There is a tendency, however, to overemphasize the importance of the lower detection limit of an assay. Of major importance is the sensitivity, defined as the ability of an assay to differentiate significantly between small differences of analyte concentrations. The sensitivity depends largely on the steepness of the calibration curve. It is highest in the steepest parts of the curve and assays usually are optimized in such a way that the diagnostically important concentration range is lying in that part of the calibration curve (Fig. 17).

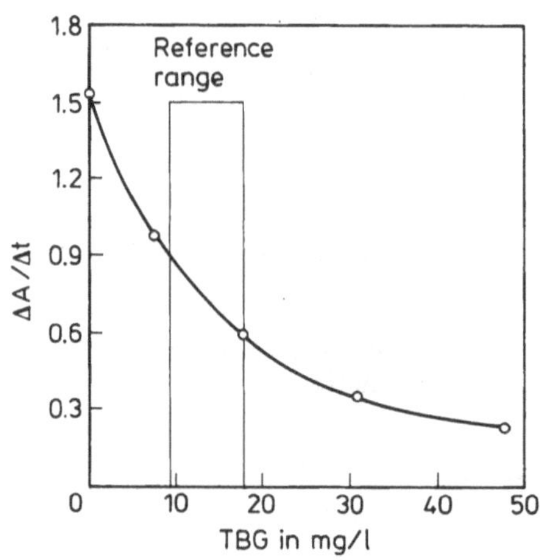

Fig. 17. Typical calibration curve of Enzymun-Test® TBG. From: Kessler, A.-Ch., Mattersberger, H. in: Methods of Enzymatic Analysis, Vol. IX, 117, Bergmeyer, H. U., Bergmeyer, J., Graßl, M. (eds.), Weinheim Verlag Chemie, 1986

3.4. Specifity

The high specificity of immunoassays is based on the hypervariable binding site regions of the immunoglobulin L- and H-chains [76-79]. Essentially 6 to 12 amino-acid residues [80,81] are responsible for the specific interaction between antigen and antibody. The chemical nature of the antigen determinant (antigenic site or epitope, terms used interchangeable) is determined by particular functional groups and their spacial arrangement [81,82].

The observation that antibodies elicited by a native protein often did not react with its denatured form [82,84] and that specific antibodies could be raised against peptides having no fixed conformation [82-84] led to the definition of two classes of epitopes: conformational (dependant on the native spacial conformation of the protein) and sequential (depending only on the amino-acid sequence of the corresponding peptide segment) epitopes. Today, however, all epitopes are seen to be conformational in the sense that the antibody-combining sites will bind only to that population of antigen conformers which presents a complementary constellation of interacting side chains: antigenic determinants are topographic, they are composed of structures on the protein surface [82].

The specificity of an EIA primarily depends on the development of the antibodies (see 4.1).

However, during the various stages of the reagent development of an enzyme-immunoassay the specficity can be altered: This may happen in the course of coupling with hapten/enzyme or coating to the solid phase. Usually these pitfalls are controlled at every step of the reagent development and in the final test protocol.

3.5 Interferences

Interferences in immunoassays have been reviewed by Nickoloff in 1984 [88] (Refs. [84]). Only some general aspects will be discussed in the following:

Nickoloff classified interferences into those common to all immunoassays (isotopic and non-isotopic) and those specific for a certain method.

Common interferences: Several immunoreactive compounds may interfere with the antigen-antibody interaction. A digoxin-like immunoreactive compound has been found in the plasma of neonate infants, in amniotic fluid, sera of pregnant women and in adults with kidney disease [89, 90]. Endogenous autoantibodies [91–97] or antibovine, antigoat, antirabbit etc. antibodies [3, 30, 98–100] may interfere with the immunoassay in rare cases.

Tubes used for sample collection may cause problems in the assay by release of the plasticizer [101, 102] or by adsorption of the analyte into the surface of the tube [103].

Specific interference factors in enzyme-immunoassays: a main type on interference is that caused by the interaction of the enzyme label and the serum matrix. Serum or plasma contains a mixture of proteins, carbohydrates, lipids, and other compounds which may serve as effectors of enzyme activity [88]. In general, heterogeneous enzyme-immunoassays will have fewer problems than homogeneous techniques, since the separation step reduces interactions with potentially interfering factors. This is why more interferences were reported with homogeneous than heterogeneous enzyme-immunoassays [88]. To avoid interference from certain serum proteins in some homogeneous assays, the serum must be pre-treated [7, 104].

3.6 Accuracy

The WHO offers reference materials for the majority of clinically interesting and immunologically detectable proteins, thus permitting calibration of the respective immunoassays. These calibration substances are primarily intended for the calibration of working (secondary) standards (e.g. national standards, or calibrators of commercial kits).

Clearly defined chemicals which can be weighed out are available for calibration purposes for virtually all of the clinically important haptens (such as T_4, digoxin, theophylline).

Definitive or reference methods do not exist for the determination of

- peptide and proteo-hormones in serum;
- haptens below serum concentrations of 10^{-9} mol/l (e.g. T_3, fT_4, aldosterone, digoxin).

Since reference methods, which could be used to check the accuracy of a given immunoassay, are not available in these cases, it is rather difficult to assess the accuracy of immunoassays in this concentration range [166].

A more limited and perhaps more realistic intermediate goal is to reach consensus values of the analyte [166]. This is why the comparability of several different commercial immunoassays has been investigated in international collaborative studies. The results from such an interlaboratory survey with TSH as analyte, performed by the New York State Department of Health as part of the endocrinology testing programme in August 1984 may serve as a typical example: Deviations from the target value varied between − 37% and +25% for individual TSH methods in the easily measurable region (around 25 µU/ml), while in the less accessible lower concentration range (target value 2.4 µU/ml) the deviation was as much as −67% to +38%.

Similarly large method-to-method differences are found with practically all tests for proteins in the concentration range below 10^{-10} mol/l (e.g. FSH, LH, insulin, prolactin, ferritin, HCH and others).

Somewhat better comparability exists for hapten tests in the higher concentration range around 10^{-10} mol/l (e.g. T_4 or digoxin). Good method comparability, particularly for hapten immunoassays, is found in the concentration range from 10^{-7} to 10^{-4} mol/l (e.g. theophylline, tobramycin, amikacin).

The poor comparability of the different types of polypeptide and protein immunoassays holds equally true for radio- and enzyme-immunoassays; the reasons are of an extremely varied nature:

- differing specificity of antibodies, e.g. in the case of CEA [105], TBG [106] and hCG [87],
- differences between the nature of the calibration material and the serum analytes (composition and origin),
- heterogeneity of the original reference material,
- matrix effects (differing influencing of the reaction by the calibrator and the matrix containing the analyte),
- type of bound/free separation technology used,
- lack of reference methods (see above).

For some time now, international organizations have been endeavouring to improve the comparability of various immunological tests. One of the possible approaches is the uniform use of human serum as solvent for the calibration material. A cortisol reference material based on human serum has recently become available from the Community Bureau of Reference of the European Community (BCR) for calibration purposes. The assigned values for cortisol were determined by isotope dilution mass-spectrometry in a native serum pool containing endogeneous and added cortisol [107].

Taking TSH as an example, a WHO/IFCC working group [108] is currently checking to see whether the use of native human serum as solvent for the WHO-TSH leads to better comparability. There are reports in the literature indicating that the use of differing solvents (bovine serum albumin, bovine serum, horse serum, chicken serum) is partly responsible for the poor comparability.

3.7 Practical Aspects and Future Developments

Homogeneous EIAs can easily be applied to a lot of mechanized analysers with incubation times of about 3 to 5 minutes [19].

Heterogeneous EIAs are more difficult to mechanize due to longer incubation periods (up to several hours) and due to the washing and separation steps. During the recent years, however, several partly and fully mechanized analyzers have become available such as ES 11, ES 22, ES 600 (Boehringer Mannheim GmbH), Stratus (American Dade), Encore (Baker Instruments Corp.) or Quantum (Abbott Diagnostics).

Great efforts are made to further improve the practicability and sensitivity of enzyme-immunoassays, notably:

— development of more sensitive homogeneous EIAs for the measurement of smaller quantities of proteins that allow easy application on routine analyzers,
— reduction of incubation times and handling steps with heterogeneous EIAs.

A rather new type of non-separation EIA has been reported by Ashihara et al. [109]. In this method a ferritin-antibody is coupled with clearly defined sites of the enzyme α-amylase. The addition of serum ferritin inhibits α-amylase from reacting with a synthetic macromolecular substrate. The enzyme activity decreases with increasing ferritin concentrations. The detection limit for ferritin in this assay is 15 µg/l. Further research has to demonstrate whether this principle can be generalized for more low concentrated proteins.

Other examples in the field of non-separation EIA are:

— determination of 5 µg/l IgG by an enzyme-channelling procedure [57],
— sensitive measurement of IgG by the "liposome technique" [113], see Fig. 8,
— determination of IgG utilizing the high affinity of the biotin-avidin complex [110],
— a horse radish peroxidase-labelled antigen was used in the determination of AFP, IgE, ferritin and β-2-macroglobulin [111].
— application of the apoenzyme reactivation immunoassay system (ARIS) for TBG- and hCG-assays [112].

So far, however, none of the above mentioned non-separation EIAs with higher sensitivity has proven its suitability in routine analysis.

The development trend in separation EIAs can be clearly shown by the example of hCG:

In 1972, the proven sandwich-EIA technique still needed a total incubation time of 4.5 hours and involved several time consuming working steps [114]. In 1986, an optimized sandwich-EIA permitted the fully automated determination of hCG on the ES 600 with a total incubation time of 90 minutes (Enzymun-Test® HCG). In the same year it became possible to carry out an hCG determination with a reaction time of just 8 minutes using a radial partition EIA [115].

Widespread use under routine conditions will show how reliably these new systems can function.

4 Components of Enzyme-Immunoassays

Enzyme-immunoassays make use of antibody, antigen/hapten, enzyme and (in heterogeneous assays) some device that allows a bound/free separation. As described in the chapter "Types of enzyme-immunoassays", these basic components are linked to each other in several ways depending on the assay employed.

4.1 Antibodies

Today's enzyme-immunoassays utilize polyclonal and monoclonal antibodies.

Polyclonal antibodies
Polyclonal antibodies still are frequently indispensable when antibodies of extremely high avidity are required.
Preparation of polyclonal antibodies: In order to avoid antibodies against impurities, the antigen should be at least 98% pure (but undesired antibodies may still occur). To obtain such purity, sophisticated purification methods must be applied, such as high performance liquid chromatography, isoelectric focusing, affinity chromatography or polyacrylamide gel electrophoreses [116]. The choice of the species to be immunized depends on the amount of antisera required and the access to laboratory animals. Preferred species are guinea-pigs, rabbits, goats and sheep. A larger animal does not need more antigen [117], repeated injections of 50–100 μg protein emulsified in complete Freund's adjuvants will give a vigorous response either in rabbits, sheep or goats.

Tests used to check the immune response are the double-diffusion method of Ouchterlony [118], the Enzyme-linked Immuno Sorbent Assay (ELISA), radioimmunoassay [119] or immunofluorescence [120].

The amount of γ-globulin G antibody in the antisera might range from 50–200 μg/ml. But exceptions up to 5–20 mg/ml can occur [121]. Due to the heterogeneity of the antisera the range of affinities can vary between 10^6 mol/l and 10^{12} mol/l [122].

With polyclonal antibodies the screening and purification procedure is very important to exclude/eliminate those antibody populations which may cross-react with similar compounds. Immunosorption procedures [123–125] and gradient elution procedures will allow the separation of antibody populations of different affinities as well as non-specific IgG binding to the absorbent matrix. To isolate TSH-specific antibodies from raw antisera of mice, immunized with TSH, for instance, the α-chain-specific ones first have to be eliminated in order to avoid interference by hCG, LH and FSH that contain α-chains with the same immunoreactivity. This separation of the α-chain immunoreactive fraction may be achieved by absorption to immobilized hCG. Only after that step can a TSH-immunosorbent be employed.

These extensive purification steps lead to high quality polyclonal antibodies with a narrow range of binding constants and high specificity [126].

Monoclonal Antibodies (Mabs)

Of great help in the improvement of enzyme-immunoassays was, of course, the discovery of monoclonal antibodies, which resolved some of the notorious problems associated with polyclonal sera (requirement of highly purified immunogens, undesirable cross-reactivity due to less specific sub-populations of antibodies, questionable reproducibility of large-scale production pools). Whenever possible, new enzyme-immunoassays therefore use Mabs, the development and purification of which has become largely routine by now.

However, monoclonal antibodies also exhibit several disadvantages:

They may show surprising properties during purification, storage and derivatization [167]. Specificity and affinity may alter under these conditions [167,168]. Due to their unique biochemical and physical properties changes of pH, ionic strength and other factors may significantly alter their physical behaviour. This is why monoclonal antibodies have been called "capricious primadonnas" [168]. Polyclonal antibodies usually react less sensitive to environmental changes, because (usually) some antibody subpopulations still will function "orderly" [136]. Because of their high specificity monoclonal antibodies usually detect exclusively only a very small fragment (epitope) of the protein. This may cause problems if that epitope shows thermodynamic lability [136]. Another commonly observed disadvantage of Mabs is the difficulty to find a population with high affinity [168].

Monoclonal antibodies are produced by immortalized, selected cell clones and are, by definition (and after careful purification), homogeneous immunoglobulins.

With this technology published by Köhler and Milstein [127] in 1975 one can produce large amounts of highly specific, homogeneous antibodies against antigens and haptens. The development of Mabs starts with the screening of sera of the immunized mice, e.g. titre, specificity, affinity and cross-reaction. Further assays have to be done during the initial screening of the primary cultures, after cloning, expansion, recloning and large-scale cultures, after ascites production and purification.

The principles of the monoclonal antibody technique are shown in Fig. 18. Spleen cells of the immunized mouse and immortal mouse myeloma cell lines are fused by polyethylene glycol. All unfused cells die in the HAT-selection medium. Hybrid cells are checked for antibody production, which is followed by cloning and propagation in the mouse of culture fluid: The culture or ascites fluid (of the mouse) contains the desired monoclonal antibody. Many detailed protocols for the production of Mabs have been published in technical papers and handbooks (see, e.g., [121,128-131]).

Specifity, avidity and binding kinetics: A very important step in the development of an immunoassay is the characterization of the monoclonal antibodies with respect to specificity, avidity and binding kinetics:

The first critical decision concerning the specificity of an enzyme-immunoassay occurs with the selection of the criteria for screening the primary culture of a (monoclonal) antibody population:

If an intact hCG molecule, e.g., is used in screening for monoclonal antibodies to hCG, three different types of monoclonal antibodies can be found [87]:

— antibodies that react only with the α-chain of hCG,
— antibodies that react only with the β-chain of hCG,
— antibodies that react only with intact hCG ("conformational antibodies").

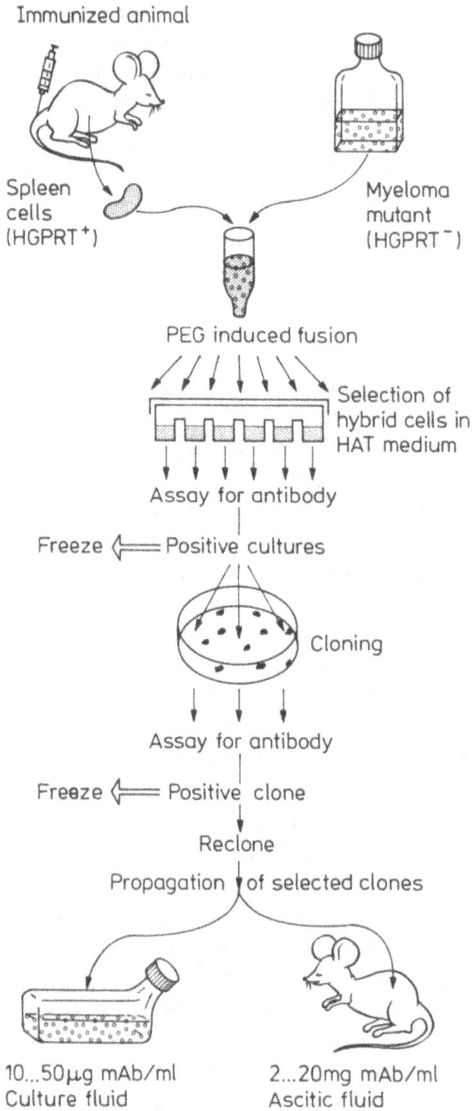

Fig. 18. Protocol for generation of hybrid cells producing monoclonal antibodies

When using this screening method, of course, no antibodies will be found, which recognize exclusively the α- or β-chain ("private" epitopes of these chains being hidden on the intact hCG), but not the hCG molecule [87].

There are a lot of methods to characterize the specificity of different monoclonal antibodies [132]. The best strategy to characterize the large variety of obtained monoclonal antibodies against a given antigen is to classify them into groups recognizing the same epitopes.

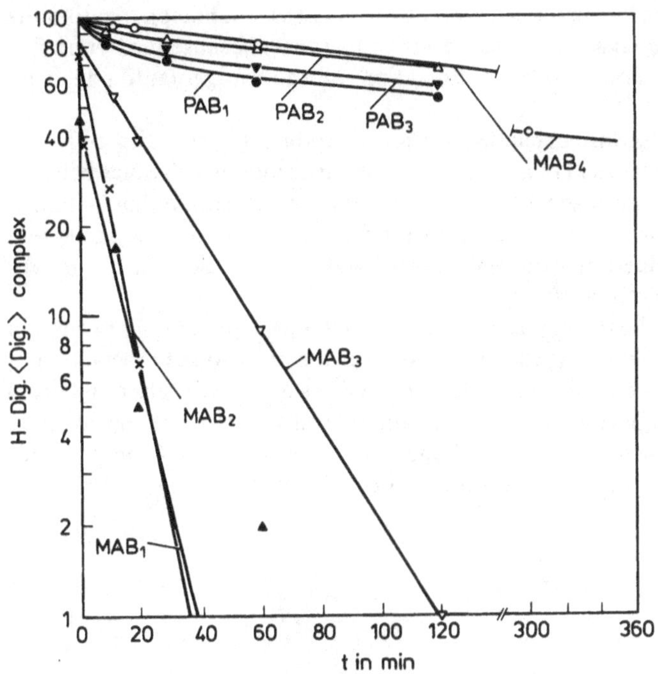

Fig. 19. Dissociation rates of several monoclonal (MAB) and polyclonal antibodies (PAB) having a similar overall high affinity to digoxin. From: Albert, H. W., in: New Technologies in Clinical Laboratory Science, Shinton, N. K. ed., 83, MTP Press Limited, 1983

One method to define the antigen binding site is based on a competitive test principle: The antigen is immobilized on a microtitre plate and a first monoclonal antibody labelled with ^{125}J or enzyme, which is known to bind to the antigen, is incubated together with a second monoclonal antibody of unknown specificity. The rate of binding of the second antibody shows the spacial relationship of the antigenic determinants, recognized by the two antibodies [133, 134]. Another type of test is a sandwich-like assay. One antibody is immobilized on a solid phase and reacted with antigen. A second labelled monoclonal antibody is tested for its ability to bind to the antigen. This is the best method to find two different groups of monoclonal antibodies which are suited for a sandwich enzyme-immunoassay [135].

Antibodies with high avidity are needed, for example, to allow sensitive assays with short incubation times. However, high avidity alone will not always be sufficient for good performance in a test system: another important feature is the velocity of the association and dissociation process. Figure 19 shows the dissociation rates of several monoclonal and polyclonal antibodies having a similar overall affinity towards digoxin. Three of four monoclonal antibodies have fast dissociation rates, whereas all polyclonal antibodies exhibit very slow dissociation rates with half-times over several hours. This finding has practical consequences in that monoclonal antibodies may be inferior to polyclonal antibodies in some test systems because the bound/free separation may cause a considerable dissociation of the antigen/antibody complex [136].

Large-scale production: Stepwise expanded antibody-producing clones can be grown in large volume cultures. The yield of antibodies in the supernatants will range between 5–10 μg/ml, sometimes it can reach 100 μg/ml medium for 10^6 cells within 24 hours. On an industrial scale hybrids are already grown in fermenters up to 1,000 l. Fermentation can replace the production of antibodies in animals, and in case of histocompatibility problems it is the method of choice.

Hybrids injected into histocompatible animals will result in tumour formation which can be enhanced by injecting the mice with pristane prior to the inoculation of the hybrid cells. The immunoglobulin levels in the ascites and the serum range from 2–20 mg/ml. For antibody purification, ion exchange chromatography is one favoured method and for IgG subclasses protein A columns can be used [162, 163]. Other methods are gel filtration and high performance ion exchange chromatography [164, 165].

4.2 Enzymes

Enzymes are used in EIAs, because the high velocity of the enzyme-substrate reaction allows the detection and quantitation of extremely small quantities of immune reactants. Enzyme activity usually is measured by photometry of chromogenic substrates. But also fluorogenic, radioactive and chemiluminescent-producing substrates are used, in order to increase the detectability of assays [19].

Ideally, enzyme labels should possess the properties listed in O'Sullivan's review [5]:

1. Availability of purified low-cost homogeneous enzyme preparations.
2. High specific activity.
3. Presence of residues through which the enzyme can be cross-linked to other molecules with minimal loss of enzyme, antibody and antigen activities.
4. Stable enzyme conjugates.
5. Enzyme absent from biological fluids.
6. Assay method that is simple, cheap, sensitive, precise, and not affected by factors present in biological fluids.
7. Enzyme, substrate, cofactors, etc., should not pose a potential health hazard.

Of course, the specific requirements for an enzyme will be dictated by the nature of the assay. For instance, in homogeneous assays and free phase IEMA-techniques the enzyme-substrate reaction should not be affected by factors present in serum samples. This requirement is not that important in separation-methods, where endogenous factors interfering with enzyme activity will be removed by the washing procedure.

A selection of some enzymes frequently used in homogeneous and heterogeneous systems is listed in Table 2 (more enzymes are cited in Ref. [5, 19]).

The properties of the enzyme conjugate are an important prerequisite for the precise measurement of the analyte over the clinically significant concentration range.

Table 2. Most frequently used marker enzymes. From: Schrenk, W. J., Kürzinger, K.: Medical Lab. Sci. *43*, 269 (1986)

Enzyme	Source	Mol. wt. (KD)	Spec. act. (U/mg)	Turnover number (min^{-1})	Reaction catalyzed in vivo	Preferred indicator reaction	Disadvantages/ Advantages
Peroxidase (HRP)	Armoracia lapathifolia (horse-radish)	40	~ 1800 (with ABTS®)	7.2×10^4	$H_2O_2 + X \cdot H_2 \rightarrow 2\ H_2O + X_{ox}$	H_2O_2 + ABTS® · H_2 → ABTS® ($\Delta A_{430-450\,nm}$)	Small, versatile glycoprotein, largely resistant to oxidants (can be coupled with periodate), but azide-sensitive.
β-Galactosidase	Escherichia coli	540	600 (with ONPG)	1.8×10^5	Lactose + H_2O → Glucose + Galactose	PNPG → p-Nitrophenol ($\Delta A_{405\,nm}$) or: 4-Methylumbelliferyl-β-D-galactoside → 4-methyl-umbelliferole	Excellent visualisation, but too large for some assay principles.
Alkaline phosphatase	Calf intestine	100	3500 (with Phe-PO_4 at 37 °C pH 9)	3.5×10^5	R-O-P + H_2O → R-OH + P_i	p-Nitrophenylphosphate → p-Nitrophenol ($\Delta A_{405\,nm}$)	Versatile glycoprotein most commonly used in sandwich assays.
Glucose oxidase	Aspergillus niger	186	210	3.9×10^4	Gluc + O_2 → H_2O_2 + Glucono-δ-lactone	Glucose → Gluconolactone; + HRP + ABTS® · H_2 → ABTS ($\Delta A_{430-450\,nm}$)	Glycoprotein larger than HRP; 2-step indicator reaction in combination with HRP.
Glucose-6-phosphate dehydrogenase	Leuconostoc mesenteroides	110	~ 700	7.7×10^4	Gluc-6-P + NADP → Gluconolactone-6-P + $NADPH_2$	NADP → $NADPH_2$ ($\Delta A_{334-365\,nm}$)	Only used in homogeneous assays.

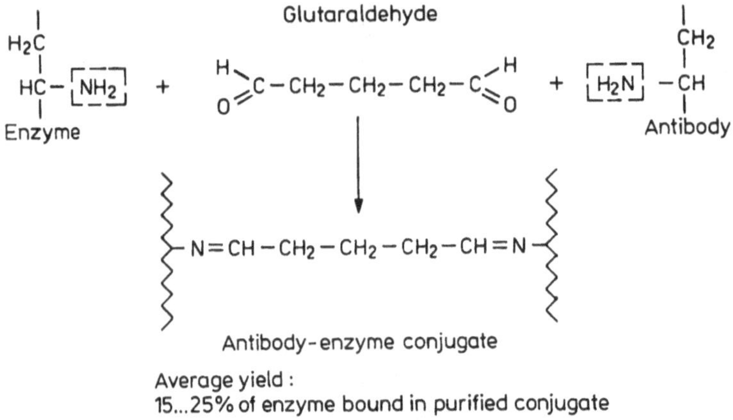

Fig. 20. 1-step glutaraldehyde method (GDA). From: Schrenk, W. J., Kürzinger, K.: Medical Lab. Sci. *43*, 269 (1986)

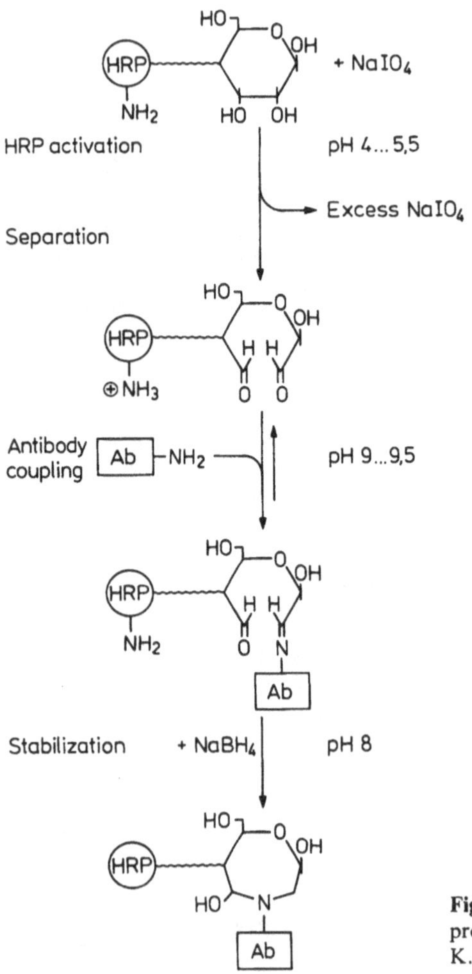

Fig. 21. Periodate method (restricted to glycoprotein enzymes). From: Schrenk, W. J., Kürzinger, K.: Medical Lab. Sci. *43*, 269 (1986)

Numerous methods have been applied to prepare protein-protein [137)] and protein-hapten conjugates [138)].

Due to the experience of the authors only conjugates between enzymes and antibodies, antigens and haptens will be discussed in the following.

4.3 Antibody-enzyme Conjugates

The main problem in linking an enzyme to an antibody is to avoid undesired cross-linking reactions caused by the cross-linking reagent. This problem is simply due to

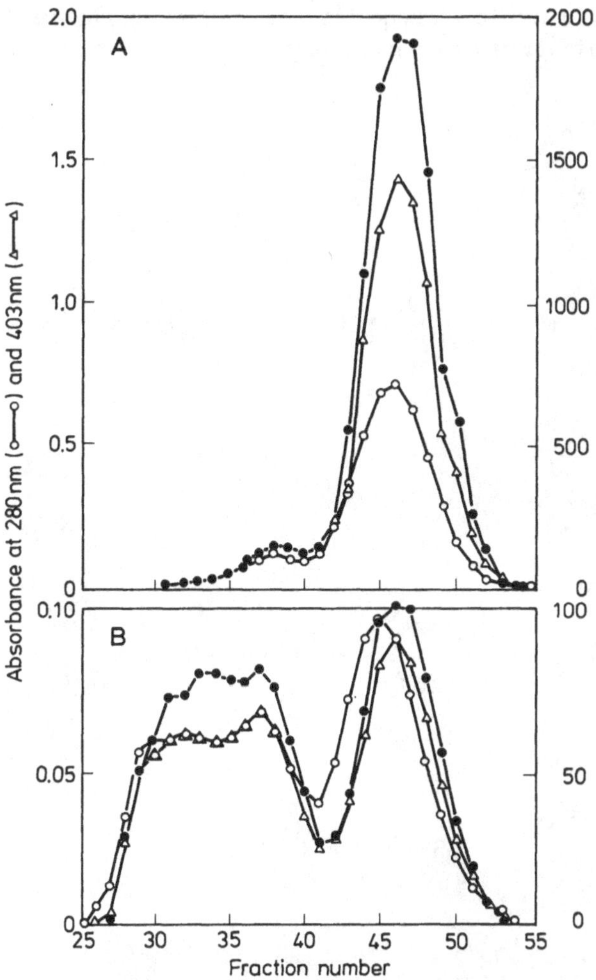

Fig. 22. Comparison of HRP conjugates obtained with the GDA (A) and the periodate (B) methods after chromatography over ultrogel AcA 44. Absorbance at 280 nm (open circles) reflects total protein concentration, absorbance at 403 nm (open squares) the heme group of HRP. Solid circles indicate HRP enzymatic activity. HRP as well as Fab' fragments remain largely unconjugated after use of the GDA method (Fig. 6A, fractions 43–52), while conjugate yield is much higher using the periodate method (Fig. 6B, fractions 26–41). From: Imigawa, M. et al.: J. Appl. Biochem. *4*, 41 (1982)

the fact that both components are proteins and contain amino acid residues with similar chemical reactivity.

For conjugation with the marker enzyme molecules, meanwhile most research groups use Fab-fragments.

The one-step glutardialdehyde (GDA)-method [139], Fig. 20 and Nakane's periodate activation of glycoproteins, i.e. HRP [140], Fig. 21, are well-established conjugation methods.

The GDA-method, however, results in a substantial loss of enżyme as well as of antibody-binding activities, whereas the periodate method gives higher yields, better binding characteristics and also a wider spectrum of conjugate molecules (see Fig. 22): yield and binding characteristics can be influenced by variation of stoichiometry (antibody to enzyme), variation of the oxidation reaction, variation of protein concen-

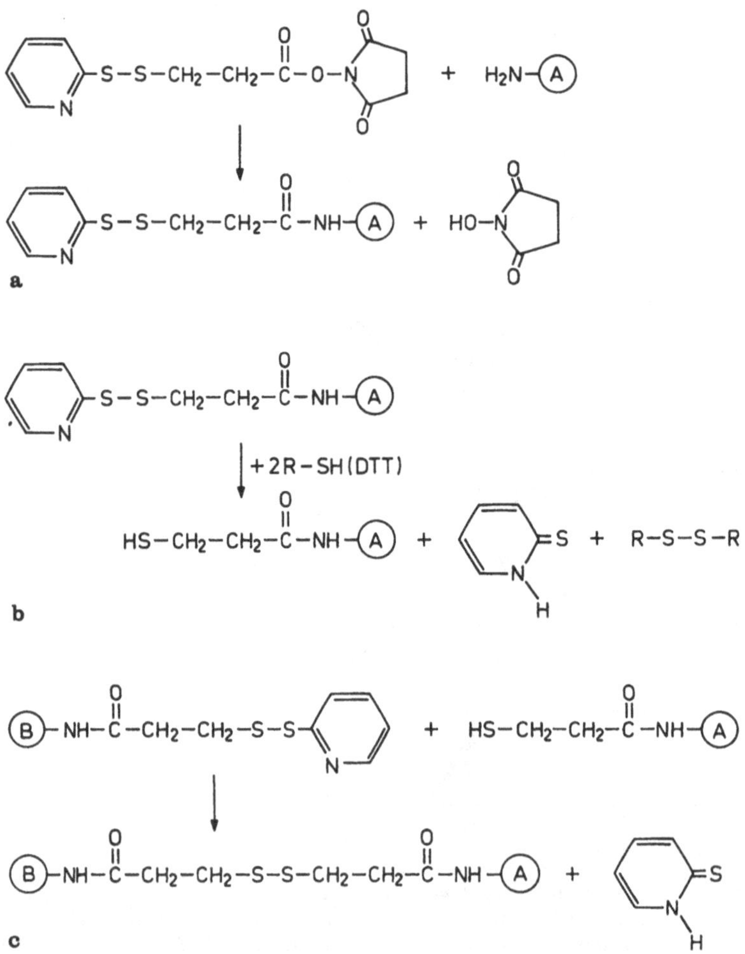

Fig. 23. Scheme for protein-protein conjugation using N-Succinimidyl-3-(2-pyridyldithio)-propionate (SPDP). From: Schrenk, W. J., Kürzinger, K.: Medical Lab. Sci. *43*, 269 (1986)

tration during the coupling reaction and of pH as well as of ionic strength. Contemporary HRP-based immunoassays usually employ only certain fractions of the whole possible conjugate range, as other may give rise to non-specific interactions with serum components or the solid phase and may have unfavourable stability, binding kinetics or sensitivity.

The use of defined organic linker molecules such as N-succinimidyl-3-(2-pyridyldithio)-propionate (= SPDP) or maleimido-hexanoyl-N-hydroxysuccinimide (= MHS) combines the advantages of both of the above methods (universality of GDA, and directed chemistry of periodate activation) while avoiding their limitations: SPDP for instance can be used with proteins in a clearly defined sequential reaction [141], Fig. 23.

If one of the reaction partners already possesses free sulfhydryl groups (e.g. β-galactosidase or F(ab')-fragments), the reaction sequence can be further simplified by employing heterobifunctional linkers of the type of MHS (Fig. 24) which are the compounds of choice to couple β-galactosidase to whole antibodies or Fab-fragments [142-144]. The reaction chemistry is mild enough to leave all biological activities

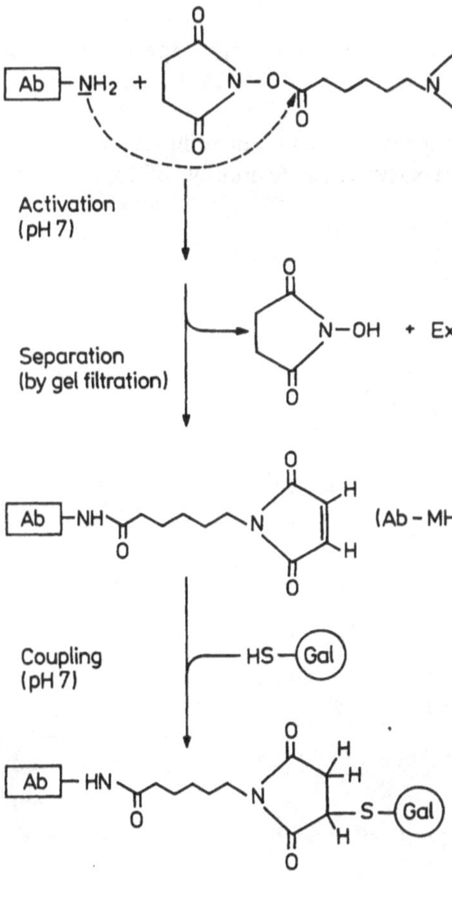

Fig. 24. Reaction sequence for conjugation of antibody and β-galactosidase using maleimido-hexanoyl-N-hydroxysuccinimide (MHS). Amino groups of intact or fragmented antibodies (Ab) are coupled to sulfhydryl groups of β-galactosidase (Gal). All steps are performed at or near neutral pH. From: Schrenk, W. J., Kürzinger, K.: Medical Lab. Sci. *43*, 269 (1986)

virtually intact; conjugate composition and size can be controlled by stoichiometry (antibody to MHS, and Ab-MH to β-galactosidase, respectively), protein concentration during coupling as well as pH and ionic strength, resulting in a large variety of products. The conjugate can be selected with respect to non-specific binding, sensitivity and kinetic performance (related to overall molecular size). For high-sensitivity immunoenzymometric assays, further conjugate purification is usually mandatory, with final yields in the range of only a few per cent of the starting antibody — which accounts for the rather high price of some of the more sophisticated commercial kits.

4.4 Antigen and Hapten Enzyme Conjugates

While the preceding paragraph has exclusively dealt with enzyme-antibody conjugates, which are needed for most of the commonly used heterogeneous EIAs such as sandwich and immunoenzymometric assays, competitive ELISAs require a different class of conjugates, i.e. between marker enzyme and analyte. If the analyte is a protein such as insulin or TBG, the coupling chemistry follows the same routes as described above. In general, the enzyme label should be small, and not to substantially alter the diffusion and binding kinetics of the derivative, making HRP the all-time favorite (Table 2) in separation methods [126,145].

This holds also true for hapten analytes, which often require highly specific methods for their activation preceding actual conjugate synthesis [146,147]. In the case of thyroxine (T_4)-HRP conjugates for example, a classical reaction of peptide chemistry is applied: a tertiary butyloxycarbonyl (BOC) group hat to be introduced in order to protect the amino function of T_4 during the subsequent formation of an activated

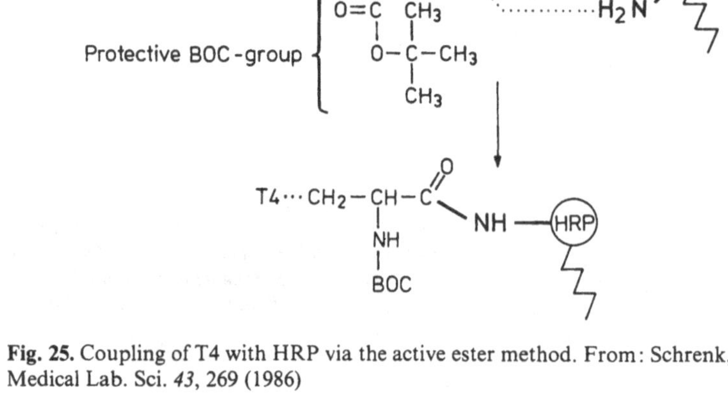

Fig. 25. Coupling of T4 with HRP via the active ester method. From: Schrenk, W. J., Kürzinger, K.: Medical Lab. Sci. *43*, 269 (1986)

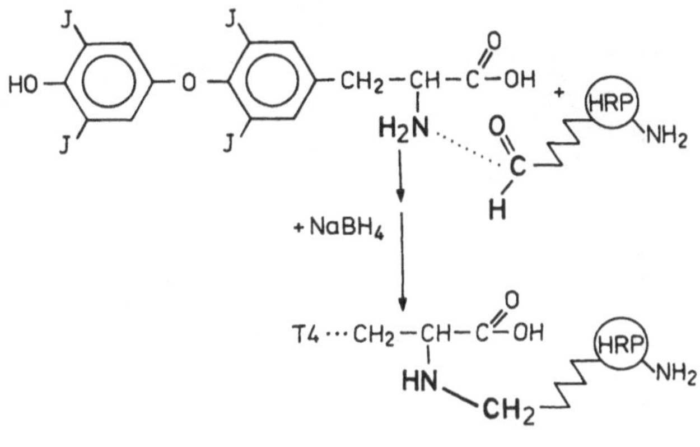

Fig. 26. Coupling of T4 with HRP via oxidation of HRP. From: Schrenk, W. J., Kürzinger, K.: Medical Lab. Sci. *43*, 269 (1986)

N-hydroxy-succinimide (OSu) ester. The protected and activated T_4 then reacts with native HRP to form stable amide bonds with the ε-amino groups of lysine residues [148], Fig. 25. In a different synthetic approach (Fig. 26), HRP is modified by oxidizing its carbohydrate moiety. The activated, aldehyde groupbearing enzyme forms a Schiff's base with the amino function of underivatized T_4. Subsequent reduction with sodium borohydride stabilizes the new linkage. Depending on the other components of the assay, especially the type of solid phase antibody used, one or the other of the two conjugates leads to superior performance, which in either case is also influenced by the stoichiometry of T_4/HPR coupling.

4.5 The Solid Phase

Contemporary separation phases are: beads of different sizes [149], magnetic particles [150], precipitates [151], fibres [152] and the inner surface of plastic tubes [9,12,30].

Either antibody or antigen is attached to the solid phase. The antibody usually is bound by a non-covalent linkage via hydrophobic forces [153-155].

It is very important that the solid phase takes up an adequate amount of the reactant in a reproducible manner. Variability at this stage probably is a major factor in determining the precision of all solid phase immunoassays [30,169].

The steepness of the dose response curve is extremely dependent on the antibody amount bound to the solid phase. Figure 27 shows a typical "binding curve" of antibody to a tube wall. Up to an antibody concentration of 1.5 μg/ml the antibody is almost completely bound to the tube wall. In the sandwich EIA Enzymun-Test® CEA finally an antibody concentration of 2.5 μg/ml in the coating solution was eventually chosen. At this concentration about 2.0 μg/ml of antibody are bound to the tube wall [156]. This excess of tube wall antibodies is an important prerequisite to having a fairly linear relationship between the optical density and the concentration of the antigen (Fig. 28).

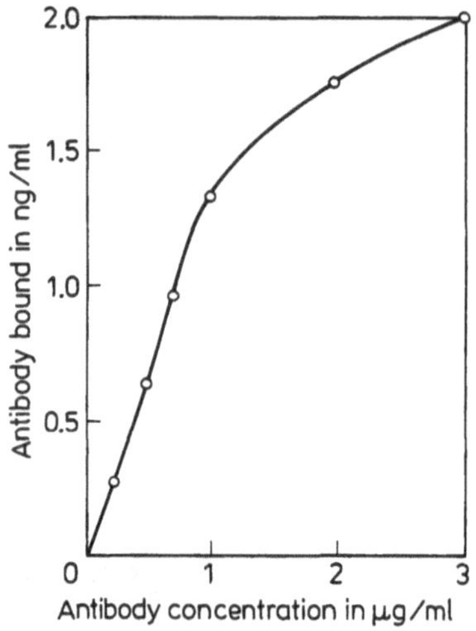

Fig. 27. Binding curve of CEA antibody to a polystyrene tube. From: Deeg, R., in: Workshop Report Enzymun-Test® CEA (156)

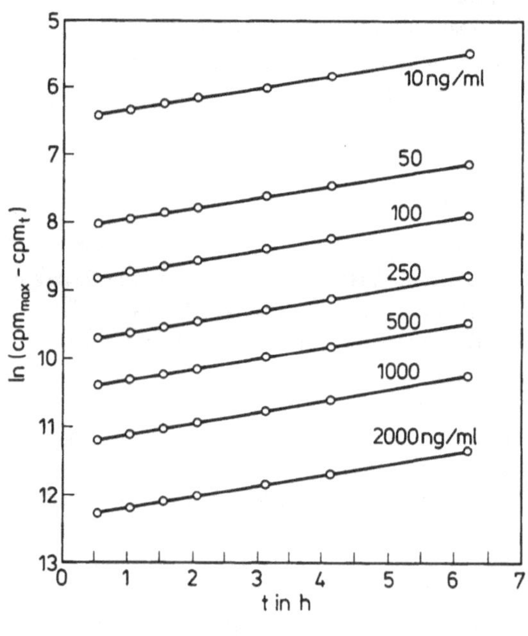

Fig. 28. Semi-logarithmic plots of ^{125}I CEA bound to antibody coated tubes versus binding time. The curves show a pseudofirst order kinetic of antigen binding to the antibody: The antigen bound to the tube wall is proportional to the initial concentration in the sample. From: Deeg, R., in: Workshop Report Enzymun-Test® CEA (156)

5 Concluding Remarks

Obviously this article could only give an arbitrary selection of examples out of the large field of enzyme-immunoassays. No end is yet in sight of the rapid progress in this area: The reliability and practicability of methods will further increase and more and more diagnostically relevant analytes will become accessible to the routine measurement in clinical laboratories.

6 References

1. Vogt, W.: Internist *22*, 308 (1981)
2. Oellerich, M.: Akt. Endokrin. Stoffw. *5*, 6 (1984)
3. Wood, W. G., Walter, D., Hantke, U.: J. Clin. Chem. Clin. Biochem. *23*, 461 (1985)
4. Sarkinnen,. H. K., Tuokko, H., Halonen, P. E.: J. Virol. Methods *1*, 331 (1980)
5. O'Sullivan, M. J., Bridges, J. W., Marks, W.: Ann. Clin. Biochem. *16*, 221 (1979)
6. Monroe, D.: Anal. Chem. *56*, 920A (1984)
7. Oellerich, M.: J. Clin. Chem. Clin. Biochem. *22*, 895 (1984)
8. Engvall, E., Perlmann, P.: Immunochemistry *8*, 871 (1971)
9. Van Weemen, B. K., Schuurs, A. H. W. M.: FEBS Lett. *15*, 232 (1971)
10. Yalow, R. S., Berson, S. A.: J. Clin. Invest. *39*, 1137 (1960)
11. Rubenstein, K. E., Schneider, R. S., Ullmann, E. F.: Biochem. Biophys. Res. Communications *47*, 876 (1972)
12. Schuurs, A. H. W. M., Van Weemen, B. K.: Clinica Chimica Acta *81*, 1 (1977)
13. Wisdom, G. B.: Clin. Chem. *22*, 1243 (1976)
14. Ngo, T. T., Lenhoff, H. M.: Appl. Biochem. Biotechn. *6*, 53 (1981)
15. Feldmann, G., Druet, P., Bignon, J., Averameas, S. (eds.): Immunoenzymatic Techniques, Amsterdam, North Holland, American Elsevier (1976)
16. Engwall, E., Pesce, A. J. (eds.): Quantitative Enzyme Immunoassay, Oxford, Blackwell Scientific Publications (1978)
17. Pal, S. B. (ed.): Enzyme Labelled Immunoassay of Hormones and Drugs, Berlin, Walter de Gruyter (1978)
18. Vogt, W. (ed.): Enzymimmunoassay — Grundlagen und praktische Anwendung, Stuttgart, Thieme (1981)
19. Oellerich, M.: Principles of Enzyme-immunoassays. In: Methods of Enzymatic Analysis (eds. Bergmeyer, H. U., Bergmeyer, J., Graßl, M.), Weinheim, Verlag Chemie, Vol. I, 233 (1983)[3]
20. Nakamura, R. M., Pito, W. R., Tucker III, E. S. (eds.): Immunoassays in the Clinical Laboratory, New York, Alan R. Liss (1979)
21. Maggio, E. T. (ed.): Enzyme immunoassay, Boca Raton, FL, CRC Press (1980)
22. Malvano, R. (ed.): Immunoenzymatic Assay Techniques, The Hague, Martinus Nijhoff (1980)
23. Ishikawa, E., Kawai, T., Miyai, K. (eds.): Enzyme Immunoassay, Tokyo, Igaku Shoin (1981)
24. Voller, A., Bartlett, A., Bidwell, D. (eds.): Immunoassays for the 80s, Lancaster, UK, MTP Press (1981)
25. Ngo, T. T., Lenhoff, H. M.: Enzyme-mediated immunoassay, New York, London, Plenum Press, p. 1 (1985)[1]
26. Averameas, S., Druet, P., Masseyeff, R., Feldmann, G. (eds.): Immunoenzymatic Techniques, Amsterdam, Elsevier (1983)
27. Talwar, G. P. (ed.): Non Isotopic Immunoassays and Their Applications, New Dehli, Vikas Publishing House (1983)
28. Butt, W. R. (ed.): Practical Immunoassay, New York, Marcel Dekker (1984)
29. Bergmeyer, H. U., Bergmeyer, J., Graßl, M. (eds.): Methods of Enzymatic Analysis, Volume IX, Proteins and Peptides, Weinheim, Verlag Chemie (1986)[3]
30. Voller, A., Bidwell, D. E., Bartlett, A.: The Enzyme-linked Immunosorbent Assay (ELISA), London, The Authors (1979)

31. Engvall, E.: Enzyme Immunoassay ELISA and EMIT. In: Methods in Enzymology, Vol. 70, p. 419, (eds.) Vunakis, H. van, Langone, J. J., New York, Academic Press (1980)
32. Clark, B. R., Engvall, E.: Enzyme-linked Immunosorbent Assay (ELISA). In: Theoretical and Practical Aspects (ed.) Maggio, E. T., p. 167, Boca Raton, CRC Press (1980)
33. Voller, A.: Heterogeneous Enzyme Immunoassays and Their Applications. In: Enzyme Immunoassay (ed.) Maggio, E. T., p. 181, Boca Raton, CRC Press (1980)
34. Grenner, G.: Principles and Applications of Heterogeneous Enzyme Immunoassays. In: Modern Methods in Protein Chemistry (ed.) Tscheche, H., p. 149, Berlin, de Gruyter (1983)
35. Müller-Esterl, W.: Practical Considerations in Enzyme-immunoassays Illustrated by a Model System, p. 15, in loc. cit. 29
36. Henkel, E.: J. Clin. Chem. Clin. Biochem. *22*, 919 (1984)
37. Esser, A. F.: Lab. Res. Methods Biol. Med. *4*, 213 (1980)
38. Olsson, T., Thore, A.: Chemiluminescence and its Use in Immunoassay, p. 113 in loc. cit. 24
39. Wood, W. G.: J. Clin. Chem. Clin. Biochem. *22*, 905 1 (1984)
40. Cais, M., Dani, S., Eden, Y. et al.: Nature (London) *270*, 534 (1977)
41. Soeni, E., Hemmilä, I.: Clin. Chem. *25*, 353 (1979)
42. Hemmilä, I.: Clin. Chem. *31*, 359 (1985)
43. Ullmann, E. F., Blakemore, J., Lente, R. K., Einstad, W., Jaklitsch, A.: Clin. Chem. *21*, 1011 (1975)
44. U.S. Patent 4.510.240
45. Burd, I. F., Wang, R. C., Feeney, I. E., Carrico, R. I., Boguslaski, R. C.: Clin. Chem. *23*, 1402 (1977)
46. Finley, P. R., Williams, R. I., Lichti, D. A.: Clin. Chem. *26*, 1723 (1980)
47. U.S. Patent 4.272.866
48. U.S. Patent 4.134.792
49. Ngo, T. T.: Int. J. Biochem. *15*, 583 (1983)
50. Morris, D. L., Ellis, P. B., Hornby, W. E. et al.: Anal. Chem. *53*, 658 (1981)
51. Tynach, R. J., Rupchock, P. A., Pendergrass, S., Kjold, A. C., Smith, P. I. et al.: Clin. Chem. *27*, 1499 (1981)
52. Sheeham, M., Caron, G., Muegler, P.: Clin. Chem. *31*, 932 (1985)
53. Lindberg, R., Ivaska, K., Irjola, K., Vanto, T.: Clin. Chem. *31*, 613 (1985)
54. Fan, S., Hedaya, E., Hwang, D., Mak, A., Malin, M., Oraivej, N., Schwarzenberg, M., Scott, M. E., Seman, K.: Clin. Chem. *31*, 909 (1985)
55. Litchfield, W. I., Freytag, J. W.: Liposomo-Entrapped Enzyme Mediated Immunoassays, p. 145, loc. cit. 25
56. Litchfield, W. I., Freytag, J. W., Adamich, M.: Clin. Ghem. *30*, 1441 (1984)
57. Litman, D. J., Hanlon, T. M., Ullmann, E. F.: Anal. Biochem. *106*, 223 (1980)
58. Zuk, R. F., Ginsberg, V. K., Honts, T. et al.: Clin. Chem. *31*, 1144 (1985)
59. Bulcke, J. A., Sherwin, A. L.: Immunochemistry *7*, 681 (1969)
60. Jockers-Wretou, E., Pfleiderer, G.: Clin. Chim. Acta *58*, 223 (1975)
61. Gibbons, I.: Nonseparation Enzyme Immunoassays for Macromolecules, p. 121, loc. cit. 25
62. Litman, D. J.: Test Strip Enzyme Immunoassay, p. 155, loc. cit. 25
63. Belanger, L., Sylvestre, C., Dufour, D.: Clin. Chim. Acta *84*, 15 (1973)
64. Carter, J. H.: Future Trends in Non-Isotopic Immunoassays, p. 11 in Syllabus, 11th Meeting Clinical Ligand Assay Society (ed.) Kolis, M., Clinical Ligand Assay Society, New Orelans (1985)
65. Masseyeff, R., Maiolini, R., Bouron, Y.: Biomedicine *19*, 314 (1973)
66. Ferrna, B., Milano, G., Ly, B., Guennec, J. Y., Masseyeff, R.: J. Immunol. Methods *60*, 257 (1983)
67. Schuurs, A. H. W. M., Van Weeman, B. K.: Dt. Ges. f. klin. Chemie e.V. Mitteilungen *10*, 22 (1979)
68. Tchen, P.: DNA *4*, 93 (1985)
69. Ngo, T. T., Carrico, R. J., Boguslaski, R. C., Burd, I. F.: J. Immunol. Methods *42*, 93 (1981)
70. Kasahara, Y., Ashihara, Y., Nishizono, I.: Clin. Chem. *31*, 912 (1985)
71. Fuhrmann, M., Graninger, W., Havel, M., Silberbauer, K.: Berichte der ÖGKC *8*, 19 (1985)
72. Oellerich, M.: J. Clin. Chem. Clin. Biochem. *18*, 197 (1980)
73. Willnow, P., Raichle, T.: Poster Scientific Bavaria (1985)

74. Meyer, H. D., Braun, S. L.: Ärztl. Lab. *31*, 308 (1985)
75. Bergmeyer, H. U., Horder, M., Markowetz, D.: Reliability of Laboratory Results and Practicability of Procedures, loc. cit. 19, 21
76. Hilschmann, N., Barnikol, H. U., Kratzin, H., Altevogt, P., Engelhard, M., Barnikol-Watanabe, S.: Naturwissenschaften *65*, 616 (1978)
77. Hilschmann, N., Craig, L. C.: Proc. Nat. Acad. Sci. U.S.A. *53*, 1403 (1965)
78. Davies, D. R., Padlan, E. A., Segal, D. M.: Ann. Rev. Biochem. *44*, 639 (1975)
79. Huber, R., Deisenhofer, J., Colman, P. M., Matsushima, M., Palm, N.: X-Ray Diffraction Analysis if Immunoglobulin Structure, in: The Immune System, 27. Coll. Mosbach 1976, p. 26, Berlin, Heidelberg, New York, Springer (1976)
80. Simon, Z.: Angew. Chem. *86*, 802 (1974)
81. Berzofsky, J. A., Schechter, A. N.: Mol. Immunol. *18*, 751 (1981)
82. Benjamin, D. C., Berzofsky, J. A., East, I. J., Gurd, F. R. N., Hannum, C., Leach, S. J., Margoliash, E., Michael, J. G., Miller, A., Prager, E. M., Reichlin, M., Sercarz, E. E., Smith-Gill, S. J., Todd, P. E., Wilson, A. C.: Ann. Rev. Immunol. *2*, 67 (1984)
83. Lerner, R. A.: Nature *299*, 592 (1982)
84. Brown, R. K., Delaney, R., Levine, L., Van Vunakis, H.: J. Biol. Chem. *234*, 2043 (1959)
85. Sela, M.: Science *166*, 1365 (1969)
86. Sela, M., Schechter, B., Schechter, I., Borek, F.: Cold Spring Harbor Symp. Quant. Biol. *32*, 537 (1967)
87. Schwarz, S., Berger, P., Wick, G.: Clin. Chem. *31*, 1322 (1985)
88. Nickoloff, E. L.: CRC Crit. Rev. Clin. Lab. Sci. *21*, 255 (1984)
89. Valdes, R. Jr., Graves, S. W., Brown, B. A., Landt, M.: J. Pediatr. *102*, 947 (1983)
90. Valdes, R. Jr., Siegfried, B.: Clin. Chem. *29*, 1166 (1983)
91. Hsu, T. H., Nickoloff, E. L., Rock, R. C., Herner, A.: J. Nucl. Med., *19*, 703 (1978)
92. Nickoloff, E. L., Hsu, T. H., Rock, R. C., Perlstein, M.: Proc. Clin. Radioassay Soc. 4th Natl. Meet., Los Angeles *28*, (1978)
93. Lipson, A., Nickoloff, E. L., Hsu, T. H.: Proc. Clin. Radioassay Soc. 4th Natl. Meet., Los Angeles *30* (1978)
94. Clayton-Hopkins, J. A., Nickoloff, E. L., Rule, A. H., Lassman, M. N., Printz, D.: Clin. Radioassay Soc. 5th Natl. Meet. Washington, D.C. *130* (1979)
95. Vidnes, A., Silsand, T., Ljosland, R., Kapelrud, H., Prydz, P. E.: Scand. J. Clin. Lab. Invest. *42*, 431 (1982)
96. Allan, D. J., Murphy, F., Needham, C. A., Barron, N., Wilkins, T. A., Midgley, J. E. M.: Lancet *2*, 824 (1982)
97. Bhagat, C. I., Garcia-Webb, P., Watson, F., Beilby, J. P.: Clin. Chem. *29*, 1324 (1983)
98. Vladutiu, A. O., Sulewski, J. M., Pudlak, K. A., Stull, C. G.: JAMA *248*, 2489 (1982)
99. Hunter, W. M., Budd, P. S.: Lancet *2*, 1136 (1980)
100. Howanitz, P. J., Howanitz, J. H., Lamberson, H. V., Benedict, S.: Clin. Chem. *26*, 1020 (1980)
101. McKiel, R. R., Barron, N., Needham, C. J., Wilkins, T. A.: Clin. Chem. *28*, 2333 (1982)
102. Shah, V. P., Knapp, G., Skelly, J. P., Cabana, B. E.: Clin. Chem. *28*, 2327 (1982)
103. Koida, M., Nakamuta, H., Matsuo, J., Yamamoto, Y., Orlowski, R. C.: Jpn. J. Pharmacol. *32*, 413 (1982)
104. Moser, R., Crompton, R. M., Scovill, D. M., Stone, A. J., Valdez, J., Centofanti, J. W., Monte, A.: Clin. Chem. *31*, 928 (1985)
105. Shiveley, J. E.: J. Clin. Immunoassay *7*, 112 (1984)
106. Kessler, A.-Ch., Rudorff, K. H., Oellerich, M., Horn, K., Mattersberger, J., Hesch, R. D.: J. Clin. Chem. Clin. Biochem. *23*, 117 (1985)
107. BCR report: EUR 99 21 EN, Marchandise (ed.) (1985)
108. WHO report: WHO/BS/85/1462 (1985)
109. Ashihara, Y., Nishizono, H., Tsuchiya, H., Tanimoto, T., Kasahara, Y.: Clin. Chem. *31*, 904 (1985)
110. Kasahara, Y., Ashihara, Y., Nishizono, I.: Clin. Chem. *31*, 912–913 (1985)
111. Hoshino, N., Hama, M., Suzuki, R., Kataoka, Y., Sol, G.: J. Biochem. *97*, 113 (1985)
112. Schroeder, H. R., Dean, C. L., Johnson, P. K., Morris, D. L., Hurtle, R. L.: Clin. Chem. *31*, 1432

113. Cole, F. X., MacDonnell, P., Myles, A., Law, S.-J., Bruman, J., Clough, K. M., Vovis, G. F.: Abstract, 2nd International Symposium on immunoenzymatic techniques, Cannes (1983)
114. DAS 2206103 (1972)
115. Product information, American Dade (1986)
116. Scopes, R. K.: Protein Purification, Principles and Practice, New York, Springer Verlag (1982)
117. Hurn, B. A. L., Chantler, S. U.: Meth. in Enzymology *70*, 104, London, Academic Press (1980)
118. Ouchterlony, O.: Acta Pathol. Mikrobiol. Scand. *32*, 231 (1953)
119. Pierce, S. K., Klinman, N. R.: J. exp. Med. *144*, 1254 (1976)
120. Nairn, R. C.: Fluorescent protein tracing, New York, Churchill Livingstone (1976)
121. Goding, J. W.: Monoclonal Antibodies: Principles and Practice, p. 250, London, Academic Press (1983)
122. Mason, D. W., Williams, A. F.: Biochem. J. *187*, 1 (1980)
123. Jaton, J. C., Brandt, D. C., Vasalli, P.: In: Immunological Methods (Lefkovits, I., Perris, B. eds.) *43*, New York, Academic Press (1979)
124. Fuchs, S., Sela, M.: In: Handbook of Experimental Immunology, Vol. I, 10. 1.–10. 6 (Weir, D. M. ed.) Oxoford, Blackwell (1978)
125. Johnstone, A., Thorpe, R.: Immunochemistry in Practice, Chat. 10, Oxford, Blackwell (1982)
126. Schrenk, W. J., Kürzinger, K.: Medical Lab. Sci. *43*, 269 (1986)
127. Köhler, G., Milstein, C.: Nature *256*, 495 (1975)
128. Galfre, G., Milstein, C.: Methods Enzymol. *73*, 1 (1981)
129. Goding, J. W.: Journ. Immunol. Meth. *39*, 285 (1980)
130. Mishell, B. B., Shiigi, S. M. (eds.): Selected Methods in Cellular Immunology, San Francisco, Freeman (1980)
131. Kennett, R. H., McKearn, T. J., Bechtol, K. D. (eds.): Monoclonal Antibodies, New York, Plenum (1980)
132. Stähli, C., Miggiano, V., Stocker, V., Staehelin, T., Härnig, P., Takacs, B.: Methods in Enzymol. *92*, 242 (1983)
133. Friguet, B., Djavadi-Ohaniance, L., Pages, J., Bussard, A., Goldberg, M.: J. Immunol. Methods *60*, 351 (1983)
134. Piechaczyk, M., Chardes, T., Cot, M. C., Pan, B., Bastide, J. M.: Hybridoma *4*, 361 (1985)
135. Kaizu, T., Kojima, K., Iwasaki, K., Yamashita, T.: Thrombosis Research *40*, 91 (1985)
136. Albert, H. W.: Monoclonal Antibodies: Advantages and Disadvantages in Production of Test system. In: New Technologies in Clinical Laboratory Science, Shinton, N. K. (ed.), p. 83, MTP Press Limited (1983)
137. Ishikawa, E., Imagawa, M., Hashida, S., Yoshitake, S., Hamagushi, Y., Ueno, T.: J. Immunoassay *4*, 209 (1983)
138. Erlanger, B. F.: Pharm. Rev. *25*, 271 (1973)
139. Avrameas, S.: Immunochemistry *6*, 43 (1969)
140. Wilson, M. B., Nakane, P. K.: In: Related Staining Techniques, Knapp, W., Holubar, K., Wick, G. (eds.), p. 215, Amsterdam, Elsevier (1978)
141. Carlsson, J., Drevin, H., Axen, R.: Biochem. J. *173*, 723 (1978)
142. Ishikawa, E., Imagawa, M., Hashida, S., Yoshitake, S., Hamaguchi, Y., Ueno, T.: Immunoassay *4*, 209 (1983)
143. Ishikawa, W., Yoshitaka, H., Yoshitake, S.: In: Enzyme-Immunoassay, Ishikawa, E., Kawai, T., Miyai, K. (eds.), p. 67, Tokyo, Igaku-Shoin (1981)
144. Kitagawa, T.: In: Enzyme-Immunoassay, Ishikawa, E., Kawai, T., Miyai, K. (eds.), p. 81, Tokyo, Igaku-Shoin (1981)
145. Porstmann, B., Porstmann, T., Nugel, E., Evers, U.: J. Immunol. Methods *79*, 27 (1985)
146. Kabakoff, D. S.: In: Enzyme-Immunoassay, Maggio, E. T. (ed.), p. 71, Boca Raton; CRC Press (1980)
147. Nambara, T., Hosoda, H.: In: Enzyme-Immunoassay, Ishikawa, E., Kawai, T., Miyai, K. (eds.), p. 106, Tokyo, Igaku-Shoin (1981)
148. Kleinhammer, G., Lenz, H., Linke, R., Staehler, F.: In: Enzymimmunoassay, Vogt, W. (ed.), p. 42, Stuttgart, Georg Thieme Verlag (1978)
149. Product Information: Abott Diagnostics, Hybritech
150. Cohen, B., Crowe, I., Craine, I., Hargitay, B., Meriadec, B., Richmann, U., Schwarzenberg, M. et al.: Clin. Chem. *31*, 909 (1985)

151. Giegel, I. L., Brotherton, M. M., Cronin, P., D'Aquino, M., Evans, S., Heller, Z. H., Knight, W. S., Krishna, K., Sheiman, M.: Clin. Chem. *28*, (1982)
152. Thunberg, A. L., Danielson, S. I., Dappen, G. M., Findlay, I. B., Sundberg, W. M.: Clin. Chem. *31*, 910 (1985)
153. Morrissey, B. W.: The Adsorption and Conformation of Plasma Proteins: A Physical Approach, in: The Behavior of Blood and its Components at Interfaces, Vroman, L., Leonard, E. F. (eds.), Vol. 283, p. 50, New York Acad. Sci. (1977)
154. Pesce, A. J., Ford, D. J., Gaizutis, M., Pollak, V. E.: Biochim. Biophys. Acta *492*, 399 (1977)
155. Cantarero, L. A., Butler, J. E., Osborne, J. W.: Anal. Biochem. *105*, 375 (1980)
156. Deeg, R.: Development of Enzymun-Test CEA, in: Workshop Report Enzymun-Test CEA, Kessler, A. C. (ed.), p. 5, Mannheim, Boehringer Mannheim GmbH (1985)
157. Würzburg, U., Heinrich, N., Lang, H., Prellwitz, W., Neumeier, D., Knedel, M.: Klin Wschr. *54*, 357 (1976)
158. Shulman, S., Mamrod, L., Gondor, M. J., Soanes, W. A.: J. Immunol. *93*, 474 (1964)
159. Grenner, G., Schmidberger, R.: J. Clin. Chem. Clin. Biochem. *17*, 156 (1979)
160. Choe, B., Pontes, J., Dong, M. K., Rose, N. R.: Clin. Chem. *26*, 1854 (1980)
161. Gerber, M., Naujoks, K., Lenz, H., Wulff, K.: Clin. Chem. *32*, 1131 (1986)
162. Ey, P. L., Prowse, S. J., Jenkin, C. F.: Immunchem. *15*, 429 (1978)
163. Goding, J. W.: J. immunol. Methods *20*, 241 (1978)
164. The Application of High Performance Ion Exchange Chromatography in Hybridoma Technology, Review, Technical Review Series, Pharmacia Fine Chemicals (1983)
165. Hill, E. A., Penney, R. J., Anderton, B. A.: Poster C 101 presented at 14th Int. Symp. on Chromatography, London (1982)
166. Masseyeff, R. F., Malvano, R.: Problems in Standardization of Enzyme-immunoassays for Antigens, p. 38, loc. cit. 29
167. Underwood, P. A., Bean, P. A.: J. Immunol. Meth. *80*, 189 (1985)
168. Falkenberg, F. W., Pierard, D., Mai, U., Kantwerk, G.: J. Clin. Chem. Clin. Biochem. *22*, 867 (1984)
169. Standefer, J. C.: Separation-Required (Heterogeneous) Enzyme Immunoassay for Haptens and Antigens, p. 203, loc. cit. 25

Author Index Volumes 1–4

The volume numbers are printed in italics

ISBN: 3-05-500379-9

FSC
www.fsc.org
MIX
Papier | Fördert gute Waldnutzung
FSC® C083411

Zeitfracht Medien GmbH
Ferdinand-Jühlke-Straße 7
99095 Erfurt, Deutschland
produktsicherheit@kolibri360.de